Why this could be the most important book in your life . . .

•

Sixty to ninety percent of visits to physicians are for conditions related to stress. The Relaxation Response counteracts the harmful effects of stress in a host of conditions including:

- Anxiety
- Mild and moderate depression
- Anger and hostility
- Hypertension
- Irregular heartbeats
- Pain
- Premenstrual syndrome
- Infertility
- Hot flashes of menopause
- Insomnia
- Irritable bowel syndrome
- And many other stress-related illnesses.

Millions have read about the Relaxation Response in *Time* magazine, *Good Housekeeping*, and *Family Circle* and have seen it described on *The Today Show*, *Good Morning America*, and *Nightline*. You can learn simple mind/body techniques to elicit the Relaxation Response without leaving home, and you can use them anywhere. The Relaxation Response is without serious side effects and reaffirms the value of prayer, meditation, and relaxation in your daily life!

A method for everyone . . .

•

"Pills, special diets, and exercises can help some people, but the Relaxation Response as Dr. Benson describes it can help everyone—healthy and not-so-healthy, strong and weak, overworked and underworked."

David W. Ewing,
Executive Editor,
Harvard Business Review

"I am delighted that someone has finally taken the nonsense out of meditation. . . . Dr. Benson gives you guidelines so that without the need to waste hundreds of dollars on so-called 'Courses,' the reader knows how to meditate—and how to adopt a technique that best suits him or herself. This is a book any rational person—whether a product of Eastern or Western culture—can wholeheartedly accept."

William A. Nolen, M.D.
author of *The Making of a Surgeon*

the Relaxation Response

by Herbert Benson, M.D.
with Miriam Z. Klipper

WHOLE CARE

AN AVON BOOK

Illustrations credits:
Figs. 1 through 6; 8; 10 through 12: Pamela Berglund, Arrco Medical Art and Design, Inc. Figs. 7; 9: Reprinted from the *Harvard Business Review*, issue of July-August 1974.

AVON BOOKS, INC.
An Imprint of HarperCollins*Publishers*
10 East 53rd Street
New York, New York 10022-5299

First WholeCare Printing: February 2000
First Avon Books Mass Market Printing: August 1976

WHOLECARE TRADEMARK REG. U.S. PAT. OFF. AND IN OTHER COUNTRIES, MARCA REGIS-TRADA, HECHO EN U.S.A.

Printed in the U.S.A.

OPM   10 9 8 7 6 5 4 3 2 1

*I am delighted to rededicate this book to Marilyn,
my wife of thirty-eight years.*

Foreword:
Twenty-fifth Anniversary Update

·

When *The Relaxation Response* was first published in 1975, the Vietnam War and the cultural upheaval that accompanied it loomed large. Only two years earlier, the Supreme Court had established a woman's right to a legal abortion in its controversial *Roe v. Wade* decision. AIDS would not be discovered for six more years. The precursor of *in vitro* fertilization, the first test-tube baby had yet to be born. Two Californians were working in their garage to build the Apple, the first mass-produced computer. Fax machines and cell phones were a gleam in their inventors' eye.

Indeed, the world today is dramatically different from the world that was first introduced to the connections of mind and body detailed in *The Relaxation Response*. Three decades ago it was considered scientific heresy for a Harvard physician and researcher to hypothesize that stress contributed to health problems and to publish studies showing that mental focusing techniques were good for the body. I broke ranks with the medical establishment when I decided to pursue this theory and to prove or disprove it in my medical research.

Today we, as a society, take for granted the multifaceted and intimate relationship between mind and body. Scientists now avidly pursue ties between brain activity and physical manifestations. Millions of Americans now elicit the Relaxation Response regularly, as Yoga classes swell, athletes report "being in the Zone," and people set up quiet places in their homes to meditate or pray.

Despite the advances that have been made, this twenty-fifth anniversary update of *The Relaxation Response* is sorely needed. Mind/body science has made enormous progress but has yet to be incorporated as an equal, fully respected partner in Western medical disciplines. As many times as science has affirmed the original message of the book over the past two-and-a-half decades, medicine and society have yet to take full advantage of the healing resources within the mind/body realm.

So much has changed: our economy is becoming more globalized, and barriers between countries are being pulled down. But we have yet to witness a corollary paradigm shift in medicine. Today, our appetites have been whetted with quick fixes, so much so that our quest for diagnostic gadgets and miracle drugs has almost overcome common sense. We expect that surgical acumen will be enough to save us and if not, the next remarkable scientific discovery will. Although mind/body therapies have been proven effective for the vast majority of everyday medical problems, we are still far more apt to run to our medicine cabinet to relieve aches and pains than to consider relaxation or stress-management techniques.

Evolution has yielded us a human body that is astonishingly reliable, able to perpetuate breath and thought, movement and experience, day after day, year after year. By and large, our bodies function even when we bombard them with stress and fatty food, even when we neglect to exercise or to get a good night's sleep. Clearly, we are blessed with an incredible internal technology.

Sadly though, we still rely far more than we should on external fixes—on medications and medical and surgical procedures developed in laboratories—and not on our natural potential for self-healing. Therapies we can purchase and caregivers we can consult, whether available through conventional or unconventional medicine, are still far more impressive to us than our own hearts and minds, lungs and hopes, muscles and beliefs, even though they sustain us day in and day out.

The Three-Legged Stool

Seeing that we continue to neglect our potential for self-healing is a source of both frustration and motivation for me. My goal has always been to promote a healthy balance between self-care approaches and more traditional approaches—medical and surgical interventions that can be magnificent and lifesaving when appropriate. However, self-care is immensely powerful in its own right. The elicitation of the Relaxation Response, stress management, regular exercise, good nutrition, and the power of belief all have a tremendous role to play in our healing.

I envision a future in which medicine is as sturdy as a three-legged stool, balanced equally by three healing resources—medications, surgery and other medical procedures, and self-care approaches. Ideally, medicine would call upon self-care for 60 to 90 percent of the everyday problems that patients experience. We would draw appropriately upon the medicines and surgeries when necessary. All three legs are mandatory.

With this future in mind, let me update you on the headway that has been made in the last twenty-five years. With a bit of history, you'll see how *The Relaxation Response* came about and what the book's findings meant to mind/body research and to the millions of people who evoke the response. You will also see how much more we must do to ensure that healing in the twenty-first century is as complete as possible.

From the Beginning

Thirty-five years ago, when I was a young cardiologist, I noticed a trend among my patients with high blood pressure, or hypertension, a silent and dangerous precursor of heart disease. Once I prescribed medications, I noticed they often complained about fainting or becoming dizzy. These were side effects of having their blood pressures lowered with medications. Patients went from feeling fine to being burdened with irritating and disabling side effects, all the result of medicine I had prescribed.

This troubled me. It appeared that by following the standard treatment approach, I was overmedicating patients—unleashing on otherwise symptomless people maddening side effects from medications that they would be required to take the rest of their lives. I soon learned that my patients were not unique. These complaints were common among people being treated for hypertension.

It was widely known that, when measured in a doctor's office, a patient's blood pressure was often higher than when it was measured by the patient himself or herself at home or in other settings. Yet the medical literature failed to explain this discrepancy sufficiently, and none of my colleagues seemed that bothered by it.

I speculated that patients exhibited falsely high levels in doctors' offices because they were nervous, and that there might be a relationship between stress and high blood pressure. Though it seems unmistakable to us today, with the clue of the word *tension* embedded in *hypertension,* no one in medicine had yet explored the correlation between stress and elevations in blood pressure even though high blood pressure was a primary contributor to the nation's *leading* cause of death.

Mind Divorced From Body

My colleagues thought I was bizarre for suggesting such a thing because we had been taught that the mind and the body were inexorably separate, as had been postulated by René Descartes, the seventeenth-century mathematician. Following Cartesian thinking, Western science never questioned this model. Except in a relatively unaccepted field of study called psychosomatic medicine, Western science had not, in the nineteen-sixties, begun to entertain the possibility that physical problems might be rooted in mental or emotional activity, or that stress as a phenomenon could engender demonstrable medical repercussions.

Nevertheless, I pursued the question. At that time I was a research and clinical cardiologist at the Harvard Medical School's Thorndike Memorial Laboratory at Boston City Hospital. I interrupted my clinical career and returned to my alma mater, Harvard Medical School, to become a research fellow in the Department of Physiology. Under the aegis of my mentor A. Clifford Barger, beloved at Harvard for his teaching skill and widely respected for his pioneering physiology research, I began investigating a connection between stress and hypertension.

We created an animal model, rewarding monkeys for increases and decreases in their blood pressure and signaling success to them with colored lights. Eventually, we were able to train the monkeys to control their blood pressure by turning on the appropriate colored lights. They regulated their blood pressure levels with brainpower alone. We published the results in the prestigious *American Journal of Physiology* in 1969.

Transcendental Meditation

Meanwhile, my findings had intrigued practitioners of Transcendental Meditation. They believed their blood pressure decreased when they meditated but had no way to document or legitimize their claims. They wanted me to study them. Since my position at Harvard was already tenuous, I initially refused the T.M. practitioners, not wanting to be associated with a group that mainstream society considered counterculture. Nevertheless, the T.M.

advocates kept insisting, and finally I decided, "Why not?" and quietly began studying them.

Robert Keith Wallace was performing similar experiments with T.M. practitioners as part of his doctoral thesis at the University of California at Irvine. After learning of each other's work, we decided to collaborate. Once the data was compiled, we found that the facts were incontrovertible. With meditation alone, the T.M. practitioners brought about striking physiologic changes—a drop in heart rate, metabolic rate, and breathing rate—that I would subsequently label "the Relaxation Response." Their blood pressures were essentially unchanged before and after meditation, but as a group, they tended to have unusually low blood pressures to begin with. Thus, their blood pressure changed only slightly during meditation. Later, we established that such low levels of blood pressure were a health benefit brought about by the regular elicitation of the Relaxation Response. I am grateful to the T.M. adherents who led me to these findings and who agreed to be studied for the benefit of medical research, regardless of the outcome.

Connections to the Fight-or-Flight Response

Amazingly, the very room and building in which my colleagues and I studied the T.M. devotees was where

Walter B. Cannon, the famous Harvard physiologist, had discovered "the fight-or-flight response" sixty years before. For those of you unfamiliar with this finding, it was revolutionary. The fight-or-flight response offered glimpses into the evolutionary momentum that equipped modern human beings with keen physiologic survival instincts. Cannon theorized that mammals have a physical ability to react to stress that evolved as a survival mechanism. When faced with stressful situations, our bodies release hormones—adrenaline and noradrenaline, or epinephrine and norepinephrine—to increase heart rate, breathing rate, blood pressure, metabolic rate and blood flow to the muscles, gearing our bodies either to do battle with an opponent or to flee.

Our studies revealed that the opposite was also true. The body is also imbued with what I termed the Relaxation Response—an inducible, physiologic state of quietude. Indeed, our progenitors handed down to us a second, equally essential survival mechanism—the ability to heal and rejuvenate our bodies. In modern times, the Relaxation Response is undoubtedly even more important to our survival, since anxiety and tension often inappropriately trigger the fight-or-flight response in us. Regular elicitation of the Relaxation Response can prevent, and compensate for, the damage incurred by frequent nervous reactions that pulse through our hearts and bodies.

Indeed, our minds need not race as they usually do but can become focused. When the mind is focused, whether through meditation or other repetitive mental activities, the body responds with a dramatic decrease in heart rate, breathing rate, blood pressure (if elevated to begin with), and metabolic rate—the exact opposite effects of the fight-or-flight response.

Essential Components

Just as the fight-or-flight response could be triggered by any number of stressful scenarios in modern life, my fellow investigators and I hypothesized that the Relaxation Response might also be elicited in a number of different ways, not just by the method espoused by Transcendental Meditation. From the T.M. technique, we extracted four essential components that would elicit the Relaxation Response:

1. A quiet environment

2. A mental device—a sound, word, phrase, or prayer repeated silently or aloud, or a fixed gaze at an object

3. A passive attitude—not worrying about how well one is performing the technique and simply putting aside distracting thoughts to return to one's focus

4. A comfortable position

Later we discovered that only the middle two components—the mental device and the passive attitude—were required. A person could be jogging on a noisy street and still elicit the Relaxation Response. The jogger needed only to maintain a mental focus and be able to return to her focus when distracting thoughts interfered. Since ancient times, diverse religious believers have said or sung repetitive prayers—practices that also elicit the Relaxation Response. Obviously, people who are nonreligious and those who do not identify with a particular religion can just as easily and routinely reap the physical rewards. In fact, the Relaxation Response could be evoked with any number of techniques—Yoga or *qigong,* walking or swimming, even knitting or rowing. The person evoking it could sit or stand, sing or remain silent.

As my colleagues and I studied the Relaxation Response, we learned that stress—and the secretions of adrenaline and noradrenaline stress produced—contributed to or caused many more medical problems than Western medicine appreciated. The Relaxation Response proved effective in treating not just hypertension but also headaches, cardiac rhythm irregularities, premenstrual syndrome, anxiety, and mild and moderate depression.

We started teaching patients to elicit the Relaxation Response in ways that were meaningful to them. In addition to the simple repetition of the word *one* suggested in this book, Catholics could recite "Hail Mary full of grace," Jewish people might say "Sh'ma Yisrael," and

Protestants might find "Our Father who art in Heaven" calming. "Isha'allah" might be repeated by Muslims, and "Om" by members of the Hindu religion. Secular or non-religious people were encouraged to focus on words, phrases, or sounds that were compelling to them, such as the words *love, peace,* or *calm.* We learned that phrases learned in childhood could be particularly powerful, evoking the calm and security felt, for example, when in the presence of loving parents and family. In this way, we observed that all types of people were able to incorporate their own belief systems and values into evoking the Relaxation Response.

How to Elicit the Relaxation Response

In my most recent book, *Timeless Healing: The Power and Biology of Belief* (Scribner, 1996), Marg Stark and I provide updated instructions for eliciting the Relaxation Response. After twenty-some years of refining my understanding of our remarkable physiologic capability, we found that the two essential steps to eliciting the Relaxation Response are:

1. Repetition of a word, sound, phrase, prayer, or muscular activity.

2. Passively disregarding everyday thoughts that inevitably come to mind and returning to your repetition.

This is the generic technique I have taught patients and that I have used myself for many years:

1. Pick a focus word, short phrase, or prayer that is firmly rooted in your belief system.

2. Sit quietly in a comfortable position.

3. Close your eyes.

4. Relax your muscles, progressing from your feet to your calves, thighs, abdomen, shoulders, head, and neck.

5. Breathe slowly and naturally, and as you do, say your focus word, sound, phrase, or prayer silently to yourself as you exhale.

6. Assume a passive attitude. Don't worry about how well you're doing. When other thoughts come to mind, simply say to yourself, "Oh well," and gently return to your repetition.

7. Continue for ten to twenty minutes.

8. Do not stand immediately. Continue sitting quietly for a minute or so, allowing other thoughts to return.

Then open your eyes and sit for another minute before rising.

9. Practice the technique once or twice daily. Good times to do so are before breakfast and before dinner.

You can also elicit the Relaxation Response while exercising. If you are jogging or walking, pay attention to the cadence of your feet on the ground—"left, right, left, right"—and when other thoughts come into your mind, say "Oh, well," and return to "left, right, left, right." Of course, keep your eyes open! Similarly, swimmers can pay attention to the tempo of their strokes, cyclists to the whir of the wheels, dancers to the beat of the music, others to the rhythm of their breathing.

A Best-Seller

The basic message of *The Relaxation Response* took little time to ignite. Within a few weeks, the book jumped to the top of the *New York Times* best-seller list. It remained on the list for months. A book about something as simple and sensible as the use of quiet, focusing techniques to calm the body went on to sell almost four million copies, to be translated into thirteen languages, and to become the self-care book most often recommended by health professionals. The book is now in its thirty-eighth printing.

Why was the book's message so revolutionary? After all, prior to the twentieth century, doctors had few scientifically proven remedies to offer patients and were forced to rely almost exclusively on the power of the mind to heal the body. That began to change when Western medicine acquired new knowledge about the human body, starting with the recognition of bacteria in the mid-1800s. Then came the discovery of insulin and penicillin in the 1920s and 1930s, the Salk vaccine in the 1950s, and an explosion of new findings in the 1960s that led to the high-tech medicine of the 1990s. When *The Relaxation Response* was published, self-care was the farthest thing from the minds of Western physicians and patients. We were still trying to get beyond the period in which patients had little but their own resources on which to rely, when the healing of serious wounds and diseases had to be left "in God's hands." Bacteria and viruses were suddenly better understood; we were enamored, and understandably so, with all the new tools medicine had to offer us—medications, surgeries, X-ray procedures, and other innovations that identified and solved problems extraordinarily well.

Mind/body medicine appeared to be unnecessary in an age when drugs could vanquish such illnesses as pneumonia and tuberculosis and when anesthesia made surgery acceptable. In 1975, medicine had almost completely dismissed the advantages of the third leg, that of self-care, thinking, "Why bother trying to take care of problems ourselves when we have such wonderful pills and procedures?" We were completely dependent on drugs and surgeries even when those techniques were not helpful, not to mention that these interventions were often accompanied by numerous side effects and escalating medical costs.

The doctor-patient relationship started to suffer as a result. Because treatments were so powerful, the medical profession believed that treatments were all that patients needed. But patients inherently understood how out-of-whack medicine was becoming, and they resented the way in which their symptoms were dehumanized. After all, physicians often reduced medical problems to test results and Latin names, and referred to a patient as "the gallstone in room 207." The focus on new tests and treatments, together with the pressures to deliver health care in a climate of ever-increasing costs, ate away at the time physicians used to talk with patients and learn about the human side of their pathology.

Bridging the Divide

It was in this climate—one of expanding reliance on technology, escalating medical costs, and slowly deteriorating doctor-patient relationships—the *The Relaxation Response* was published. In many ways the book cast a rope across a widening chasm. In simple, scientific terms, the book—based on research my colleagues and I had published in medical journals—spelled out connections between the mind and body that were reasonable and meaningful to both Western scientists and their patients. They suggested that mind and body were not as diametrically opposed as our culture had decided they were.

With that first rope thrown across, we could now bridge a gulf. East and West might be joined; science and the everyday experience of human beings could be brought together in meaningful ways. In many instances, that is what occurred. The chasm was crossed, the gulf bridged. However, true progress—the recasting of perspective in traditional medicine—was far more plodding than I had hoped. My work and that of my colleagues had already helped many people, which was a source of great satisfaction for me. On the other hand, many more could have been helped, and we might have had a far greater therapeutic impact on both patients and on the costs of patient care, if the academic medical community had been as enthusiastic as the public was about our findings.

The Public's Enthusiasm

Within weeks of the book's publication in 1975, I traveled to New York from my home in Boston and was astonished to find copies of my book heaped on the front table at a Fifth Avenue bookstore. After all, I had been surprised to be asked to write a book in the first place. Bill Adler, an agent who represented authors as famous as Howard Cosell, had called me to suggest that my research would make an interesting book. However, neither of us could have predicted the public reaction to *The Relaxation Response* or the trends in book publishing it began, predating a slew of subsequent medical best-sellers by Bernie Siegel, Norman Cousins, Deepak Chopra, Andrew Weil, Dean Ornish, and others.

Barbara Walters played a major role in the success of *The Relaxation Response* by interviewing me on ABC's *Good Morning America.* Sitting backstage after the show, I remember having to set aside the medical students' exam papers I was grading to teach Ms. Walters to elicit the Relaxation Response as she had asked me to. I was so invested in what Harvard academics thought of my work that the media attention embarrassed and worried me.

It also didn't occur to me that the national media attention would have an impact on my life. I could not have imagined that people who read *The Relaxation Response* would become its staunchest supporters and fervent publicists. The book helped hypertensive people lower their blood pressure, eased the pain of those with migraines and other aches and pains, and gave people more reasons to pray. Because of the profound impact *The Relaxation Response* had on their lives, strangers greeted me at speaking engagements as if I was a treasured friend.

I counted on the objective scientific proof of the research my associates and I performed to bring about a profound change in medicine—in which the influence of the mind was as tenaciously investigated by researchers as the influence of drugs and technological gains. I believed the three-legged stool model would be incorporated; drugs, surgeries, and self-care would be used equally and appropriately. I had no idea this alteration of medical practice would be such an uphill battle.

Only the Placebo Effect

The argument most frequently used to disregard our findings was the suggestion that the Relaxation Response was nothing more than the reobservation of the prevalent—and I might add, consistently misunderstood—placebo effect. In other words, critics said that the physiologic changes my colleagues and I observed in our clinical patients were self-suggested or "all in the patients' heads." By believing they could lower their blood pressure, patients had been able to do so. In other words, belief in the Relaxation Response was responsible for its success. People got better simply because they imagined themselves better.

Yet, that much was true in all scientific experiments on humans. Researchers had long known that when patients believed they would get better—when, for example, they believed they were taking medicine but were instead taking placebos such as sugar pills—more than 30 percent of them did actually improve. Randomized control trials were first extensively used in Western medicine after World War II, when massive new drug experiments were launched. It was then that the placebo effect became an irritating component of scientific experiments, a kind of black sheep in medicine.

I had as much disdain for the placebo effect as my colleagues, so I worked diligently to prove the Relaxation Response was a distinct physiologic state. I read hundreds of scientific studies, examining how the placebo effect had entered into medical developments of every kind.

Together with other researchers, I established that the success of the Relaxation Response was not attributable to the placebo effect. The Relaxation Response worked regardless of a patient's belief. Indeed, when a person focused his or her mind and returned to the focus when interrupting thoughts occurred, a set of measurable, reproducible, and predictable changes occurred in the body, meeting the standards of scientific medicine. The placebo effect, by contrast, was not predictable or reproducible.

In our study, however, we found that the placebo effect was 50 to 90 percent successful, working two to three times more often than it should have, according to the 1955 report of one of my Harvard teachers, Henry K. Beecher. My colleagues and I published articles about this in 1975 in the *Journal of the American Medical Association* and in 1979 in *The New England Journal of Medicine*. Ironically, the placebo effect from which I had been so eager to distance the Relaxation Response, turned out to be a valuable and neglected asset in medicine.

Researchers had long relied on the 30 percent success rate attributed to the placebo effect by Dr. Beecher. Our work showed that far from an irritating little variable, the placebo effect deserved our utmost attention. Indeed, evolution made it an innate capacity for healing within each of us—a resource that could be effective the majority of the time. To disassociate it from the negative response it provoked in medicine, I proposed renaming it "remembered wellness." Remembered wellness, the placebo effect, is fueled by belief.

The Faith Factor

In my practice, I found that belief—and for many, this might mean religious beliefs—could not be divorced from the medical experience, as traditional medicine required. Belief was central to patients' lives, and potentially central to their health.

Eighty percent of my patients chose prayers as the focus of their elicitation of the Relaxation Response. For this reason, I found myself in a curious position—that of a physician teaching patients to pray. By no means had I set out to do this. Patients' religious affiliations were as diverse as their ages and medical conditions, but they demonstrated to me the role that religious belief could play in healing.

Remembered wellness (the placebo effect) appeared to enhance the effectiveness of the Relaxation Response. I called the combined force of these two internal influences "the faith factor," and discussed them more fully in my subsequent books, *Beyond the Relaxation Response* and *Timeless Healing: The Power and Biology of Belief*.

Philanthropist Laurance S. Rockefeller took an interest in the faith factor and the role that belief, especially religious belief, could play in all types of healing, and he sponsored our seminars for clergy from all denominations. Clergy members took the message of the faith factor back to their faith communities, where believers could benefit from the healthful effects of the Relaxation Response and remembered wellness. The renowned investor Sir John Templeton invited me to become an adviser to the John Templeton Foundation, where I encountered many other physicians, physicists, clergy people, historians, and future planners—all of whom were devoted to studying the pervasive power of God and religious belief.

I am deeply indebted to both these men, whose support ensured that my colleagues and I would gain a far greater understanding of religious faith, belief in healing, and spirituality than we would have otherwise.

Fear of mixing church and state, religion and science, is predominant in our culture. My colleagues and I tried to avoid this controversy altogether, simply by offering our patients a choice. When teaching patients to evoke the Relaxation Response, we asked them, "Would you prefer a secular or religious approach?" We enabled patients to bring their religious beliefs, which are often profound, into medical settings and yet we did not offend patients who did not consider themselves religious. We put patients at ease, allowing them to choose a self-tailored approach. And patients were far more apt to adhere to a regular practice of mental focusing if the approach they selected was meaningful and compelling to them personally.

The Next Fifteen Years

Many different groups, from churches to corporations, from spas to professional associations, began to clamor for the information my colleagues and I disseminated in medical journals, lectures, training sessions, and in the subsequent books we wrote. Interest in what the brain could do for the body was so intense that we frequently could not keep up with requests for speaking engagements. We could not develop programs fast enough for health care professionals, clergy, and schoolteachers. Thousands of patients sought help at our clinics.

Academic medicine, on the other hand, largely dismissed our findings for the next fifteen years. Many people were helped because I had published a best-selling book, but in many ways, that same situation hurt our cause of changing Western scientific thinking. Its very popularity tainted it in academic circles and prevented its message from being taken seriously. To my knowledge, there had never before been a best-selling author among the Harvard Medical School faculty. I was, in fact, admonished, "Physicians at Harvard do not write popular books."

To this day, physicians who become best-selling authors in this country often leave academic medicine. But I stayed at Harvard because I enjoyed its unique intellectual environment. Besides, I felt I should remain in such an academic setting to introduce real change into medicine. No matter how eager popular culture was to embrace mind/body research, Harvard and the nation's other leading teaching hospitals and research institutions were the gatekeepers of medical innovation. Harvard's prestige and reputation, which it richly deserves, would carry mind/body medicine farther than the fading glory of best-selling books.

Alternative Medicine

Practitioners of alternative medicine were eager to welcome me into their fold because they believed our work afforded them scientific credence. Most other people, in fact, lumped our findings together with "alternative medicine," believing that any approach other than pills or procedures must be "alternative." Many people believe that the only true medicine is that which can be given to you or performed upon you. Even though the elicitation of the Relaxation Response was a scientifically proven method of healing, it did not fit the traditional model of pills and procedures that Western society considers "medicine."

Throughout my career, I resisted being associated with alternative medicine. I did this for several reasons.

First, our findings were evidence-based and subjected to the strict standards of Western scientific medicine. I contend that a treatment or technique ceases to be "alternative" once it has survived the battery of scientific proofs and has been published in peer-reviewed medical journals. Alternative treatments such as herbs and homeopathy would no longer be considered "alternative" if they were evidence-based, if they met the three standards of scientific medicine—measurability, predictability, and reproducibility.

Second, a major asset of the Relaxation Response and remembered wellness is that they are self-administered.

Their power lies within each of us. In this way, self-care is revolutionary and quite different from the medicine commonly practiced in both traditional and nontraditional settings. After all, alternative medicine, in large part, also relies on drugs and procedures, the same approaches that Western medicine overuses. Their approaches to healing are imposed on you, not evoked from within. I believe that mind/body medicine has yet to be totally accepted by both traditional *and* alternative medical communities.

Third, alternative medicine adds costs to traditional medicine while the Relaxation Response and other self-care approaches reduce costs. Research has shown that when mind/body medicine is employed, patients make fewer visits to their doctors at health maintenance organizations. In prepaid, capitated organizations such as HMOs, this is money in the bank. The nation stands to save billions of dollars each year, simply by incorporating mind/body approaches into medicine. Billions more out-of-pocket dollars could also be saved if patients did not feel compelled to pursue alternative treatments.

I believe that patients' extensive use of alternative medicine results largely from their beliefs in different therapies and the fact that their needs are not well met by traditional medicine's reliance on the first two legs of the stool—pills and procedures. After all, doctors today spend seven or eight minutes with a patient, on average, whereas alternative practitioners average thirty minutes with each patient.

Also, alternative medicine fits the accepted model of having a treatment done "to you." We think every medical problem requires dramatic action. Rather than cultivating and nourishing the internal healing properties within our bodies, patients place their faith in caregiver after caregiver, pill after pill, procedure after procedure, first traditional then nontraditional.

In truth, both conventional and alternative medicine owe some of their effectiveness to the placebo effect, or remembered wellness. A patient's belief that aspirin will help his headache contributes to its success the same way it would contribute to the success of an herb he took if he believed that it would alleviate his headache. Since the placebo effect is 50 to 90 percent effective, the odds are in his favor that whatever method he chooses will help, because he believes that it will. Indeed, you and I often impose beliefs on the medicines that we receive, which helps them work.

The main difference between conventional and alternative medicine is that most conventional treatments will work for the ailments for which they are appropriate, whether or not you believe in them. You do not have to believe in penicillin for it to work. A cataract transplant will restore your sight whether or not you believe it will. This is the essential difference between evidence-based and unproven, alternative methods. One works without the influence of remembered wellness, the other does not.

The National Institutes of Health and its National Center for Complementary and Alternative Medicine are now exploring the unproven claims practiced in nontraditional medical settings. I encourage this exploration, but I believe even more strongly in further investigating and employing an already proven strategy—the very powerful healing resources within each of us that can be self-administered.

A Fine Line

As you can see, I have walked a very fine line over the course of my career. I have been accepted by many and rejected by others whose opinions I valued. I have had to balance two roles at the same time, that of a traditional academician and that of a researcher and spokesperson for a new and controversial field of medicine.

As intrigued as I was by mind/body medicine, I knew it was unwise at first to associate myself solely with such a controversial field. I remained a cardiologist, chairing medical school courses and committees, while simultaneously pursuing my mind/body research. It was not until 1988, when my colleagues and I founded the Mind/Body

Medical Institute at the Deaconess Hospital, that I was able to devote my energies to the work I truly loved.

My double life meant that I published my findings in respected medical journals. Yet, I also remained committed to writing books for the public so that lay-people had access to the wonderful new information my colleagues and I were uncovering about mind/body connections.

For many years, I also could not bring myself to "practice what I prescribed." I did not elicit the Relaxation Response myself, as beneficial as I knew it could be for my body. I worried that by eliciting the Relaxation Response, I would be considered nonobjective, or a "true believer." Only when I began to experience the aches and pains that come with age did I say, "Enough is enough," and begin to follow the advice I had given others for two decades.

Nevertheless, I continued to take full advantage of the triage of healing therapies available within medicine's repertoire. In fact, several years ago, I needed medical interventions to save my life. I had an accident, having foolishly mounted an unstable chair in our kitchen to attach draft-preventing plastic to an air-conditioning vent. The chair slid out from under me, hurling me onto the edge of a butcher-block table. I broke five of my ribs. My lung was punctured and collapsed, and it caused my chest cavity to fill with blood and fluid, making it difficult for me to breathe. Had it continued unabated, the pressure would have led to the collapse of my other lung and to my death.

Luckily my wife was there to call 911 and to have me transported to the nearby Lahey Clinic. The diagnosis was made and a tube inserted into my chest. The blood and fluid were drained, my lung expanded, and my life sustained. No amount of mental focusing or other self-care would have helped. I needed this surgical procedure. This procedure, like so many that snatch people from the throes of death, ensured my existence the way nothing else could.

After this experience, I can personally vouch for the necessity of a balance between caregiver-administered and self-administered treatment. Exercise, stress management, the elicitation of the Relaxation Response, and the beliefs I had in my own recovery quickened my healing. However, my healing would never have been possible without the immediate and dramatic intervention of medical professionals.

Advanced Meditation

Having become fascinated with the health benefits of simple meditation, I wanted to study advanced meditation as well. After all, if simple meditation could be so transforming, might advanced practices be correspondingly powerful? Yet, true practitioners of advanced meditation, the Tibetan monks for example, were initially uninterested in scientific validation or in being studied.

I was persistent, however, and met with the Tibetan monks' leader, His Holiness the Dalai Lama, first in 1979 at Harvard and a dozen times after that. We became friends, discussing the fascinating ways in which the monks' practice of ancient religious rites and our team's research overlapped. In the 1980s, my teammates and I repeatedly traveled to Northern India and studied Tibetan monks who were living there in exile. There, our team witnessed incredible mind/body feats. Monks, in little clothing, remained alive and well, practicing an advanced form of meditation in temperatures of zero degrees Fahrenheit at altitudes over fifteen thousand feet in the Himalayan mountains.

In another example, the team watched as monks, dressed in nothing but small loincloths, were draped in wet sheets while exposed to near-freezing temperatures. You and I would experience uncontrollable shivering, develop hypothermia, and perhaps die under these circumstances. But because these monks had developed amazing physiologic control over years of practicing this type of heat-producing meditation, they experienced no distress in these conditions. Instead, within minutes, the body temperatures they produced steamed and dried the wet, cold sheets.

The monks accomplished this first by meditating and evoking the Relaxation Response in the same simple way my colleagues and I had studied. When their minds were quiet, they then visualized a fire or heat that came "from the scattered consciousness of the universe" and traveled through an imagined central vessel of the body. They believed this fire burned away the "defilements of improper thinking."

Eager to reproduce, in some measure, the benefits we had witnessed in the Tibetan monks, my colleagues and I from that point on began to teach our patients the "two-step process" the monks had practiced. First, you evoke the Relaxation Response and reap its healthful rewards. Then, when your mind is quiet, when focusing has opened a door in your mind, visualize an outcome that is meaningful to you. If you are intent on alleviating a pain, envision yourself without the pain. If you are concerned with your performance at work or on the golf course or tennis court, imagine yourself performing well in these venues. Whatever your goal, these two steps can be powerful, allowing anyone to reap the benefits of the Relaxation Response and take advantage of a quiet mind to rewire thoughts and actions in desired directions.

The Latest Findings

In pursuit of a balanced medical approach, my collaborators and I treated thousands of patients and published scores of studies in medical journals. One by one, we have identified medical conditions that can be relieved or altogether eliminated with the help of the Relaxation Response, remembered wellness, and other self-care approaches such as exercise, stress management, and nutrition. We learned that with self-care, we can effectively treat any disorder to the extent that it is caused by stress or mind/body interactions. Indeed, we can partly relieve or cure most of the common complaints patients bring to their doctors' offices, simply by applying self-care techniques. By taking advantage of the cost-free, healing resources within all of us, the United States, by conservative estimates, stands to save over $50 billion in wasted health care expenditures each year.

Here is a list of conditions that, to the extent caused or affected by mind/body connections (such as stress and the fight-or-flight response), can be significantly improved or even cured when self-care techniques are employed:

- angina pectoris
- cardiac arrhythmias
- allergic skin reactions
- anxiety
- mild and moderate depression
- bronchial asthma
- herpes simplex (cold sores)
- cough

- constipation
- diabetes mellitus
- duodenal ulcers
- dizziness
- fatigue
- hypertension
- infertility
- insomnia
- nausea and vomiting during pregnancy
- nervousness
- all forms of pain—backaches, headaches, abdominal pain, muscle pain, joint aches, postoperative pain, neck, arm, and leg pain
- postoperative swelling
- premenstrual syndrome
- rheumatoid arthritis
- side effects of cancer
- side effects of AIDS

Recently we pursued a greater understanding of mind/body medicine at work by studying another religious group and their practice of spirituality-based healing. Christian Scientists are known to eschew medications and treatments as part of their religious tradition. We worked with the Gallup International Institute to compile and contrast data about hundreds of Christian Scientists and non–Christian Scientists chosen randomly across the country. We concluded that the church's practitioners report far more use of spiritual practices and fewer instances of illness, and that they are more satisfied with their lives than non–Christian Scientists. Although Christian Scientists report similar numbers of doctors' visits and hospitalizations to non–Christian Scientists, they use prescription medications far less. These findings led us to conclude that a combination of routine medical treatments and mind/body approaches could offer profound health benefits.

How to Use Self-Care

Every illness has a mind/body component and some potential for benefit if you employ self-care techniques. But how do you determine the appropriate use of the advice in this book for your particular medical problem?

Always start by discussing your medical complaint with your personal physician. That way, when appropriate, you can be sure to take advantage of the drugs and procedures we are so fortunate to have. If you have tension headaches, mind/body techniques can be used to eliminate them, without the use of pills or procedures. But if you have pneumonia, you need antibiotics. And if you have cancer, you need all three legs of the stool, all the resources medicine can offer you. That is why it is critical to inquire about a health problem or concern, first and foremost, with your physician. That way, all three of these very valuable tools can be used for your care.

If you see your doctor and are disillusioned because there appears to be no medical therapy for your condition, if the physician yields you little time, or if you believe in unconventional therapies, you may consider alternative medicine. If you do take this course, you may be helped. Remember, however, that your *belief* in the treatments may very well be the major contributor to your healing. You might save the money by recognizing your own ability to produce wellness—by evoking the Relaxation Response and other self-care methods.

Fear and Guilt

Many of us are truly frightened by the notion of having control over our own health. We prefer to hand control over to doctors and alternative practitioners, and to rely on their prescriptions and directions rather than adopting healthier habits and more balanced lives ourselves. We prefer to have a named medical condition that can be treated, no matter how serious, than to have mind/ body symptoms that might be benign.

Take the case of a woman who went to many physicians with vague symptoms of on-again, off-again weakness and numbness that appeared first in one area of her body, then in another. Doctors had told her, "It's all in your head," at worst making her condition sound like a figment of her imagination and at best suggesting that her body was responding to stress she must be experiencing in her life.

Finally, another doctor did an extensive work-up and found that the woman had an incurable disease that would eventually cause death. Yet, when the doctor informed her of this, the woman said, "Oh, I'm so relieved, I thought it was all in my head." In fact, she was so concerned that she was being judged a hypochondriac, being called "mentally disturbed," and that physicians were giving up on her, leaving her helpless, that she preferred a serious diagnosis.

Our thinking is backward in this respect. What a powerful message we send our bodies when we try repeatedly to present doctors with symptoms that are treatable only with drugs and procedures. As a society, we lend medicine too much power over us, searching for answers outside of our bodies, when they may lie within us. In fact, patients who practice self-care and take control of their health become so empowered that they recognize how much medicine and society need the paradigm shift I've described.

On the other hand, it is injurious to give too much weight to mind/body interactions. Must those of us diagnosed with cancer or heart disease believe we brought these conditions on ourselves? If we cannot beat these insidious diseases, does it mean we are not strong enough in character and beliefs to turn our health around? The guilt associated with this way of thinking is enormous.

Guilt is not necessary. Employ a balanced approach. There is no proof, for example, that mind/body interactions cause cancer although they may affect its course. Place mind/body therapies within a proper context. They are but one of many influences and treatments. If diagnosed with cancer, for example, use mind/body interactions, but also use chemotherapy, surgery, and radiation. Then, whatever happens, you can rest assured you have done everything that was possible. You will have left no stone unturned.

The Paradigm Shift Underway

Every day, more and more health professionals seem to appreciate the vast potential of mind/body connections. I feel blessed to have discovered the Relaxation Response and subsequently to have realized the power of remembered wellness at a relatively young age.

A full third of Americans regularly practice a technique that elicits the Relaxation Response. In 1975, only 7 percent of Americans did so. Back then, meditation and other mind/body approaches were largely considered counterculture and extreme. Today, mind/body techniques and the practice of nourishing one's spirit are mainstream concepts.

How wonderful it was in the 1990s to have peers begin to traverse the chasm, to swing from the ropes over the artificial divide between mind and body that we are systematically taught. In 1992, an endowed Harvard professorship, the Mind/Body Medical Institute Professorship, was established in honor of our work. This professorship will be named after me upon my retirement. Wonderfully, courses about mind/body medicine and spirituality are now an established part of the curricula in most medical schools everywhere, and are some of the most sought-after classes among aspiring physicians.

In 1995, we achieved another scientific milestone. The National Institutes of Health, the world's leading source of medical research funds, devoted a "Technology Assessment Conference"—a prestigious assemblage of experts—to assess relaxation and behavioral approaches. They concluded that relaxation techniques should be incorporated into the treatment of all forms of chronic pain.

And, in 1999, the federal government, based in part on testimony I gave before the U.S. House of Representatives and the U.S. Senate in 1998, appropriated $10 million to the National Institutes of Health to create Centers for Mind/Body Interactions and Health across the country. The Centers will conduct mind/body research and training. The Senate Fiscal Year 1999 Appropriations report states:

> . . .*The Committee recognizes that stress contributes to a host of medical conditions confronted by health care practitioners, and current pharmaceutical and surgical approaches cannot adequately treat stress-related illnesses. Mind/body approaches, particularly those of the relaxation response and those related to utilizing the beliefs of the patients, have been used successfully to treat these disorders. The Committee is aware that the Mind/Body Medical Institute at the Harvard Medical School is at the forefront of research on mind/body interactions and their clinical applications. The Committee is encouraged by the results of this research and the health and cost benefits of mind/body approaches. The Committee encourages OBSSR [Office of Behavioral and Social Sciences Research] to establish pilot mind/body medical centers to make more visible the benefits of mind/body medicine; to expand its scientific base; and to teach and train health care professionals in these approaches. . . .*

I am very proud of this outgrowth of our work, the establishment of these Centers, which will markedly expand the research database and could lead to self-care treatments being further incorporated into medicine.

Even though two-thirds of physicians now recommend

mind/body approaches to their patients, the medical community has yet to achieve the balance of the three-legged stool. Medicine continues to be a reductionist practice, determined to find specific factors that cause an illness as well as specific pills and procedures that alleviate it. While this approach has great merit, changes do not occur in the body in isolated steps. Rather, many steps take place simultaneously. Mind/body interactions are a perfect example. And self-care is multidisciplinary, involving everything from nutrition to stress management, outlooks, values, and beliefs—habits of a healthy lifestyle that work together and do not fit the isolated treatment model.

Health insurance reimbursements are often based on the reductionist model. Health-care providers are reimbursed for specific pills and surgeries but not for multidisciplinary self-care treatments. How ignorant it is for these companies to ignore the data and neglect the potential benefits and cost savings of mind/body techniques.

Furthermore, academic medicine has institutionalized certain edicts that make change very difficult. For example, the criteria of scientific protocols that are used by editors of medical journals correctly require that control groups of patients embarking on an experimental therapy must be matched with groups that receive placebo treatments. However, the groups are not truly matched unless their beliefs and expectations are taken into account. Mind/body medicine teaches us that different beliefs can produce different results. Therefore, if the power of a subject's beliefs is fully acknowledged, it would invalidate many previous research studies and explain why many times, medical studies fail to be replicated. The effects of our beliefs could explain the contradictions.

The Mind/Body Medical Institute

For our part, the Mind/Body Medical Institute will continue to document the ways in which the Relaxation Response, belief and remembered wellness, stress management, exercise, nutrition, and other aspects of self-care can make major contributions to the health of all people. We'll continue to bridge the chasm, bringing potent mind/body interactions together with the other resources caregivers can administer.

The Mind/Body Medical Institute has become a model for the world, as it embraces the potential of self-care techniques. There are now fourteen affiliates nationwide, all of them teaching patients and health professionals a more balanced approach to care. The Mind/Body Medical Institute is also ensuring that the next generation understands the value of self-care far better. By introducing the Relaxation Response in schools at elementary, junior and senior high school levels, and at universities, as championed by M. J. Wilcher, we help young students cope with life's stresses in more constructive ways.

We hope that someday every doctor-patient relationship will have a mind/body component to it, both in the diagnosis and treatment of the problem. Every encounter we have with our health care professionals should take into account the effect of our beliefs, anxieties, and hopes on our health, not only because the economics of medicine will demand it but because patients look to physicians to speak to their souls as well as their ailments. Science has brought us this far, revealing the startling powers of both mind and body. My hope is that science will bring us farther still, shifting the paradigm, teaching us to use the tremendous gifts we have to heal ourselves. In so doing, vast amounts of money can be saved. What a wonderful prescription of health, happiness and prosperity for our minds and bodies, as well as our nation's economy!

Words of Thanks

Over the years most of my colleagues have been women and I owe them a debt of gratitude. Our research has shown that women more readily understand and call upon mind/body principles in their lives and in their health. This may be the reason why women patients were often mistreated and labeled "hysterical" in the past.

Again, our society promotes this backward thinking. Instead of hailing the insights of mind/body medicine that women more readily understand, male physicians often denigrated what we did not understand or could not measure. Our research has impressed upon me that women are born with and maintain an especially active link between their beliefs and their physiology, between their emotions and their health.

Female physicians, a large influx of whom entered medicine's ranks in the 1970s, 1980s and 1990s, welcomed mind/body research back into the fold of medicine where it belonged. I believe that as more of my female colleagues assume leadership within academic medicine, they will usher the principles of self-care into the next millennium.

I'd like to thank other colleagues, friends, and family members as well. I was fortunate to have been indoctrinated into medicine by instructors who cared deeply about the bedside manner, who taught me that reaching out and helping people was what medicine was about, and who supported me in my fledgling and controversial career. Robert H. Ebert, Lawrence B. Ellis, and Mark D. Altschule were among an older tradition in medicine, back when doctors took time to listen to patients and enlist their motivation in promoting health. These wonderful mentors encouraged me to make my findings widely known. Together with philanthropists William K. Coors, Laurance S. Rockefeller, Arman Simone, and John M. Templeton, they ensured that our fullest understanding of the Relaxation Response, of faith and belief, and remembered wellness would develop.

My dear friend and colleague Richard Friedman joined the staff in 1986. Friedman specialized in clinical and experimental psychology and mind/body research but he was also a champion of the Institute's cause, a man who encouraged all of us to see the impact we were having beyond Harvard, the forest beyond the trees, if you will. Richard goaded us to communicate our findings more broadly, saying, "The scientific world is getting the message. You may not know it yet but you are making great progress." Before his untimely death two years ago, Richard saw the scientific community begin to turn around and recognize the mind/body connections to which he had contributed so much. In fact, Richard's contributions were acknowledged in a three-page article in *Science,* an unusual amount of space in such a mainstream scientific journal. This pleased him tremendously.

I am even more indebted to my family. Though a few of my colleagues thought I was crazy from the beginning, I would surely have become so if it were not for the stability offered me in family life, in nearly four decades of marriage, and in raising and listening to two children. My wife and I are now blessed to be grandparents as well.

In closing, I want to thank Marg Stark for her superb help in writing this update.

For more information about the Mind/Body Medical Institute, to purchase our audio- or videotapes, to inquire about our training programs, or to find out if there is an affiliated Institute near you, visit our website at *www.mindbody.harvard.edu.*

Twenty-five years ago, this Web site address would have been gibberish, the words *Web site* not even in our lexicon. Who knows? Maybe the next twenty-five years will render it gibberish once again. And, by 2025 and beyond, medicine and surgery will be markedly different. I am confident, however, that one thing will not change. The immense, transforming power of the mind and body, of our beliefs, and of self-perpetuated healing will remain within us—eternally.

Herbert Benson, M.D.
Boston, Massachusetts
2000

1

.

An astute physician is lamenting the times:

"But the present world is a different one. Grief, calamity, and evil cause inner bitterness . . . there is disobedience and rebellion . . . Evil influences strike from early morning until late at night . . . they injure the mind and reduce its intelligence and they also injure the muscles and the flesh."

This chronicler lived 4,600 years ago in China, even though his observations appear contemporary. Human beings have always felt subjected to stress and often seem to look longingly backward to more peaceful times. Yet with each generation, complexity and additional stress are added to our lives. The truth is that most of the persistent problems of this planet are even further from solution than when the Chinese doctor decried them. The technology of the past forty-six centuries, and especially that of the last century which was supposed to make life easier for people, often seems to intensify the stress in our day-to-day existence.

Victims of Stress

What psychological price do we pay in attempting to adjust to the knowledge that war or its imminence is with us every day? Are we proud that our scientific know-how has increased the sophistication of weapons since that time when a shepherd named David could defeat an entire army with a rock thrown from a sling? Or do we knowingly or subconsciously despair of the current nuclear weaponry that could exterminate every human being, indeed almost all life?

Most of us find that we are helpless in solving the big problems. We have some vague hope that the leaders we elect (and the experts they in turn rely on) can find the solutions. But our concern usually involves everyday difficulties. Our frustrations come about because we generally can't even solve the less earthshaking problems, such as being on time to work in a large, congested city. Indeed, the everyday demands of living make it more and more difficult to escape the increasingly adverse psychological effects that seem built into our existence. Whatever it may be—the daily commute, or the rising cost of living, or the noise and fumes of the city, or unemployment, or random violence—we find it difficult to reach a satisfactory equilibrium, and as a result we become the victims of stress.

Our rapidly changing world has necessitated many other adjustments. For example, before the women's-liberation movement had filtered so far and deep, people were married under a set of unspoken agreements that society now questions and sometimes shatters. Today, women must reexamine their own roles and life-styles against conflicting expectations and suppositions. For the older woman, the problems of reeducation and readjustment can be overwhelming. Men must also adjust to a new role that may mean more responsibility for family and household. They are being forced to view women in a new way, one that may be threatening to their accustomed role. Concurrent with and related to the movement is the change of the family structure. Mobility separates families into small nuclear units. Women raise children outside of marriage. Divorced fathers assume custody of children. All share in the impact of societal changes.

How are these anxieties and stresses affecting us? The presence of mental stress as a part of modern living has been the subject of a number of books, most of which concentrate on the psychology of stress. We will consider stress from a somewhat different perspective, for our concern is not only the psychology but also the *physiology* of stress. We will explore what happens to you internally under stressful situations and how stress *physically* undermines your health. This will be done by examining the relation between your emotional reactions and what they may cost you in hypertension, heart attacks, strokes, and other diseases. We will then point out what you can do about the effects of stress. We will show how, by your personal adoption of a simple psychological technique, you can improve your physical and mental well-being.

The Hidden Epidemic

We are in the midst of an epidemic, one that is all too prevalent in the United States and other industrial nations. The name of this epidemic is hypertension, the medical term for high blood pressure. Hypertension predisposes one to the diseases of atherosclerosis (hardening of the arteries), heart attacks, and strokes. These diseases of the heart and brain account for more than 50 percent of the deaths each year in the United States. Therefore, it is not surprising that various degrees of hypertension are present in 15 to 33 percent of the adult population. Although this epidemic is not infectious in nature, it may be even more insidious, simply because its manifestations do not affect large numbers at the same time and because we are not generally aware that the disease is slowly developing within us. Throughout its course there are few, if any, symptoms. Yet each day we see it strike without warning, cutting short by decades the lives of our friends and loved ones. According to carefully compiled Government vital statistics, the diseases resulting from this epidemic account for an average of two deaths every minute in the United States alone. Put another way, that is nearly one million out of two million deaths a year. Translate this statistic into your own personal experience—the loss of a friend who leaves young children, the premature death of a father about to enjoy his retirement years. You are a fortunate individual if you have not personally experienced the ravages of this epidemic.

High blood pressure, heart attacks, and strokes have markedly increased, not only afflicting a growing percentage of the population but steadily finding their way into younger age groups. The late Dr. Samuel A. Levine, an eminent American cardiologist, pointed out in 1963 that in families he had treated for many years, sons suffered heart attacks at an average of thirteen years younger than the age at which the fathers experienced theirs. Today many cardiologists observe this same significant shift. Five to ten years ago it would have been a relatively rare event to witness a stroke or heart attack in a person in his thirties and it would have been astonishing if the patient were in his twenties. Now interns and house staff just starting in medicine consider heart attacks in men in their thirties commonplace.

There is no shortage of theories to explain the rapidly increasing prevalence of hypertension and the associated increase in the number of heart attacks and strokes, suffered mainly in the Western world. The traditional explanations have been (1) inappropriate diet, (2) lack of exercise, and (3) family disposition. Yet there is another factor, which has often been ignored: environmental stress. Although environmental stress is gaining recognition as an important factor in the development of these diseases, it is still poorly understood. All four factors play a role. What has yet to be adequately determined is the relative significance of each.

Doctors have recognized for years that stress is taking a toll. It is not difficult to understand the correlation between the highly competitive, time-pressured society in which we live and mental stress with its influence on heart disease. For example, a commonly heard warning is "Don't get upset, you'll get high blood pressure." The problem has been how to quantify stress. In other words, how do we objectively measure the effects of stress upon the body? Medicine has recently made inroads, moving from psychological speculation to hard, measurable, physiologic data.

Our focus will be on the relation between stressful psychological events and their associated physiologic changes, as they affect your health. Traditionally, psychology and medicine have long been separated by their different methodologies of research. This dichotomy has kept most physicians from seeing the relation between the psychologically laden term "stress" (hinging as it does on personal behavior and environmental events) and the functioning of the body and related diseases. Although most doctors would agree that stress does affect health, they are not attuned to the psychological, nonmedical literature about stress. Concerned mainly with bodily signs and symptoms, the physician treats stress by prescribing medication and, when no specific diseases are present, by reassurance and counseling. More often than not he will dispense so-called tranquilizing drugs rather than delve into the psychological roots of the problem. On the other hand, most psychiatrists and psychologists do not directly treat organic disease states. Their major concerns are emotions, thoughts, and personality. Psychiatrists may prescribe pills, but treatment is directed essentially to the psyche. If bodily symptoms are apparent, the patient will most likely be referred to a medical doctor, thus completing a circle with little interplay between the professions.

However, these traditional barriers are slowly crumbling. There is still a long way to go, and most physicians, because of the very paucity of concrete data, remain distrustful of psychosomatic or psychophysical diagnosis and treatment. Nevertheless, the specialty called psychosomatic medicine, which is the study and treatment of diseases caused or influenced by psychological events, is now a rapidly spreading field of medical research.

The Fight-or-Flight Response

The stressful consequences of living in our modern, Western society—constant insecurity in a job, inability to make deadlines because of the sheer weight of obligations, or the shift in social rules once binding and now inappropriate—will be described here in a manner that clearly explains how they lead to the ravaging diseases such as hypertension which are prevalent today and which are likely to become more widespread in the years ahead. We are all too familiar with the stresses we encounter. However, we are less knowledgeable about the consequences of these stresses, not only psychological but physiologic. Humans, like other animals, react in a predictable way to acute and chronic stressful situations, which trigger an inborn response that has been part of our physiologic makeup for perhaps millions of years. This has been popularly labeled the "fight-or-flight" response. When we are faced with situations that require adjustment of our behavior, an involuntary response increases our blood pressure, heart rate, rate of breathing, blood flow to the muscles, and metabolism, preparing us for conflict or escape.

This innate fight-or-flight reaction is well recognized in animals. A frightened cat standing with arched back and hair on end, ready to run or fight; an enraged dog with dilated pupils, snarling at its adversary; an African gazelle running from a predator; all are responding by activation of the fight-or-flight response. Because we tend to think of man in Cartesian terms, as essentially a rational being, we have lost sight of his origins and of his Darwinian struggle for survival where the successful use of the fight-or-flight response was a matter of life or death.

Man's ancestors with the most highly developed fight-or-flight reactions had an increased chance of surviving long enough to reproduce. Natural selection favored the continuation of the response. As progeny of ancestors who developed the response over millions of years, modern man almost certainly still possesses it.

In fact, the fight-or-flight response, with its bodily changes of increased blood pressure, rate of breathing, muscle blood flow, metabolism, and heart rate, has been measured in man. Situations that demand that we adjust our behavior elicit this response. It is observed, for example, among athletes prior to a competitive event. But the response is not used as it was intended—that is, in preparation for running or fighting with an enemy. Today, it is often brought on by situations that require behavioral adjustments, and *when not used appropriately, which is most of the time, the fight-or-flight response repeatedly elicited may ultimately lead to the dire diseases of heart attack and stroke.*

If the continual need to adjust to new situations can bring on a detrimental fight-or-flight response, and if we live continuously with stressful events which trigger that response, it is natural to question whether we know how to check the dangerous results that inevitably follow. Take this line of reasoning one step further. If the fight-or-flight response resides within animals and humans, is there an innate physiologic response that is diametrically different? The answer is Yes. Each of us possesses a natural and innate protective mechanism against "overstress," which allows us to turn off harmful bodily effects, to counter the effects of the fight-or-flight response. This response against "overstress" brings on bodily changes that decrease heart rate, lower metabolism, decrease the rate of breathing, and bring the body back into what is probably a healthier balance. This is the Relaxation Response.

★   ★   ★

This book will first explain the ways in which heart attacks and strokes develop within the body, often undetected, through the insidious mechanism of high blood pressure. We will show how high blood pressure is related to stress through the inappropriate elicitation of the fight-or-flight response.

Our main purpose, however, is to discuss the Relaxation Response, for it may have a profound influence on your ability to deal with difficult situations and on the prevention and treatment of high blood pressure and its related, widespread diseases including heart attacks and strokes. The Relaxation Response has always existed in the context of religious teachings. Its use has been most widespread in the Eastern cultures, where it has been an essential part of daily existence. But its physiology has only recently been defined. Religious prayers and related mental techniques have measurable, definable physiologic effects on the body which will be explained. From the collected writings of the East and West, we have devised a simplified method of eliciting the Relaxation Response and we will explain its use in your daily life. You will learn that evoking the Relaxation Response is extremely simple if you follow a very short set of instructions which incorporate four essential elements: (1) a quiet environment; (2) a mental device such as a word or a phrase which should be repeated in a specific fashion over and over again; (3) the adoption of a passive attitude, which is perhaps the most important of the elements; and (4) a comfortable position. Your appropriate practice of these four elements for ten to twenty minutes once or twice daily should markedly enhance your well-being.

2

•

If you owned a factory and a sales representative called on you to sell you a "miracle" machine that would never fail to distribute vitally needed materials to all points of your plant, you'd probably give him a few minutes of your time. When he told you this machine was designed to last over seventy years and pump more than two and a half billion times, indeed, circulating between forty and eighty million gallons of essential "fuel" to keep your factory functioning, you might begin to doubt that such a fantastic device really could exist.

Yet every living man and woman in the world possesses just such a machine, the human heart. The pressure generated by the heart is called blood pressure. Like any other machine, however excellent, the heart is subject to defects. High blood pressure, when the heart beats too forcefully, is one such defect. High blood pressure is so widespread in our society that it afflicts between twenty-three and forty-four million Americans.

Statistics, however, do not explain what is happening to cause high blood pressure, or hypertension, and how hypertension actually leads to heart attacks and strokes. We will first explain several basic biologic and medical principles, which will give you an adequate background to understand these events.

Vital Functions

High blood pressure, or hypertension, is very dangerous because it increases the rate of development of what is technically called atherosclerosis, commonly known as hardening of the arteries. The popular name is well chosen. Atherosclerosis is the deposition of blood clots, fats, and calcium within the walls of the arteries, causing the normally soft, elastic, open arteries to become hard, inelastic, and partly or completely blocked (see Figure 1). This blockage leads to dire consequences. But, before we

NORMAL

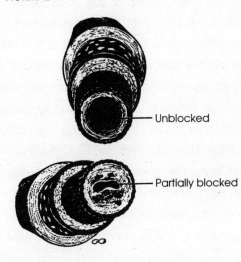

ATHEROSCLEROTIC

Figure 1
Normal, unblocked artery compared to partially blocked atherosclerotic artery.

discuss atherosclerosis, several basic principles of how the body functions should be understood.

The arteries perform a key function. They carry the blood from the heart, the pump of the body, to the body's many functional units, the cells. Tissues are simply a specialized group of cells with a common function. Different groups of tissues with a special function are organs. For example, the heart is an organ made up of muscle and other types of tissue. The function of the heart is to pump blood. The blood is another tissue. In the blood, carried by the arteries and other blood vessels, are the foodstuffs and vital components that keep the tissues alive, such as digested proteins, carbohydrates, fats, and other necessary nutrients, as well as vital oxygen. Each cell slowly "burns" its nutrients with oxygen to derive usable energy and maintain life.

Early in evolution most organisms were unicellular, made up of only one cell, living in what we would now call the sea. It was simple for these organisms to get nutrients for survival. They took them from the surrounding sea and excreted their wastes into this large reservoir by a type of simple passage called diffusion (see Figure 2). As forms of life became multicellular and more complex, the cells were removed from a direct source of nutrients. Cells became surrounded by other cells, and nutrients and wastes could no longer make their way in and out of cells by diffusion. A circulation was necessary to carry the environment of the sea to the individual cells of the body (see Figure 3).

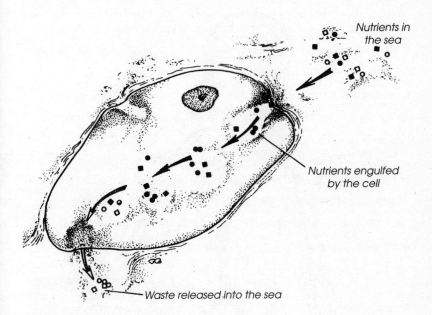

Figure 2
A single cell surrounded by the sea.

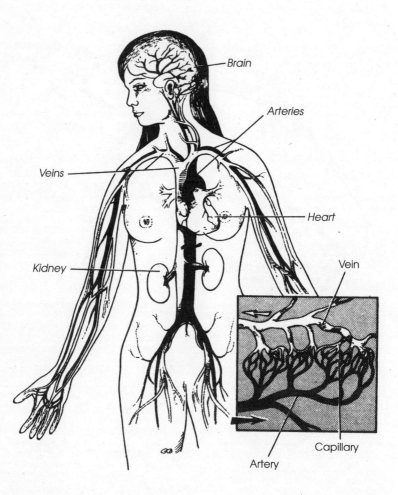

Figure 3

A diagram of the circulation, showing the blood vessels (the arteries and veins) and the following organs: the brain, the heart, and the kidneys. The insert shows the tiny vessels, the capillaries, which connect the arteries to the veins.

Our blood is part of that hypothetical sea. The circulation of the blood carries food particles from the digestive organs, such as the small intestines, and oxygen from the lungs to the cells. Special organs such as the kidneys developed to eliminate waste products, carried to them by the blood, which could no longer be eliminated by diffusion directly into the sea. In this circulatory system, the vessels that carry the nutrients from the heart to the tissue are the arteries; the veins, on the other hand, return the blood to the heart and lungs. The tiny vessels connecting the arteries and veins are the capillaries (see Figure 3). The capillaries are very thin-walled. It is through the thin-walled capillaries that the blood and the cells exchange nutrients and waste products (see Figure 4). The capillaries and the rest of the circulatory system transmit the "sea" to the cells so that they can maintain life.

The propelling force within the blood vessels is expressed as the blood pressure, which is measurable and can be described in numerical terms. It should be within relatively definable normal limits so that the tissues will receive adequate blood. To determine "normal" blood pressure, investigators measured populations' blood pressures and arbitrarily defined "normal" as where more than 90 percent of the blood pressures happened to be. When outside these limits, blood pressure is either abnormally high or abnormally low.

If blood pressure is extremely low and the heart is not

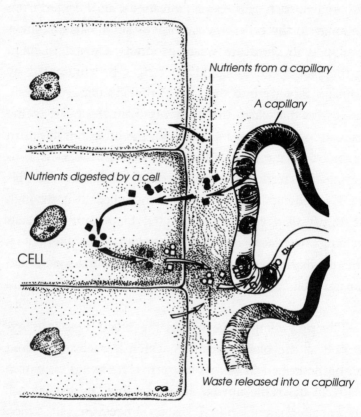

Figure 4

A cell within the body surrounded by other cells. The cell is pictured receiving nutrients from and releasing wastes into a small blood vessel of the circulation—a capillary.

pumping effectively, the tissues will not receive adequate blood supply and nutrients, and a state of "shock" will result. Ten or fifteen years ago, low pressure *per se* was considered a bad thing. For example, many young women were thought to suffer symptoms of weakness and fatigue because their measured blood pressures were low and they were given drugs to raise their blood pressures to an arbitrarily determined higher level. Today, however, it is believed that the lower the blood pressure, provided there are no adverse symptoms such as marked dizziness and fainting, the better off and the more protected you are from the ultimate development of atherosclerosis.

The risk of developing atherosclerosis or hardening of the arteries is directly related to the level of blood pressure. When you have a higher blood pressure, the risk simply increases. The higher your blood pressure, the greater the risk. The lower the better. Thus, normal blood pressure is difficult to define, although arbitrary limits have been established.

Further complicating the concept of a "normal" blood pressure is the rise and fall of blood pressure at different times of day. Blood pressure is an extremely fluctuating physiologic function. Thus, when you are actively exercising or emotionally upset your blood pressure is higher than when you are resting quietly or sleeping. But when your blood pressure is elevated above what is considered normal for most of the day, you are considered to have high blood pressure. This relatively persistent high blood pressure increases the risk of developing atherosclerosis and its related diseases, heart attacks and strokes.

Most visits to a doctor include having blood pressure measured. When a doctor measures blood pressure, he or she is measuring the blood pressure within an artery, usually an artery within the arm. A cuff is wrapped around your arm and a bulb squeezed so that the cuff becomes tighter and tighter (see Figure 5). Inside the cuff is a closed bladder made of rubberlike material which inflates with air. When the bulb is pressed, air is being pumped into that bladder, steadily increasing the pressure to very high levels and ultimately collapsing the underlying artery (see Figure 5*a*). A stethoscope is then placed over the artery to listen for sounds. Gradually air is let out of the bladder. When the pressure in the bladder falls below the pressure in the artery, a squirt of blood will come through the artery (see Figure 5*b*). This motion of blood set into action, a turbulent squirt, creates a sound, and this first sound is recorded as your highest component of blood pressure—systolic blood pressure. The sounds continue as long as the artery is constricted by the cuff (see Figure 5*c*). When the cuff no longer restricts the flow of blood in the artery, the sounds due to the turbulence totally disappear (see Figure 5*d*). The pressure at which sounds disappear or are altered is considered the diastolic blood pressure, the lowest component of blood pressure.

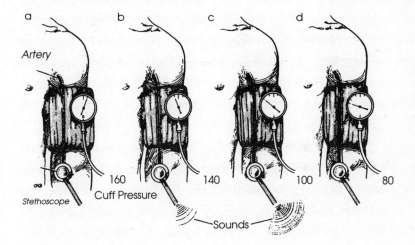

Figure 5

A diagram of how blood pressure is measured. In *a*, the pressure in the cuff is so high at 160 that the underlying artery is blocked and no sounds are heard through the stethoscope. In *b*, when the pressure within the cuff is diminished to 140, a squirt of blood comes through the artery and a sound is heard. In *c*, as the cuff pressure is diminished squirts of blood come through the still partly constricted artery, and sounds are still heard. In *d*, at a cuff pressure of 80, the artery is not constricted, blood flows through the artery in an unrestricted fashion and the sounds disappear or are altered. The blood pressure of the subject pictured is 140 systolic (the highest component of blood pressure), 80 diastolic (the lowest component of blood pressure), or 140/80.

Normal circulation is vital to maintaining a healthy internal milieu. Deprive a cell, tissue, or organ of its nutrients and it will die. For example, deprive it of oxygen and it cannot survive, because oxygen is necessary for the cell's normal functioning and use of energy, called its metabolism. If the arteries to the heart, or coronary arteries, are obstructed, then you experience death of heart cells and what is called a heart attack or a coronary or an infarction (see Figure 6).

Strokes may occur in much the same way. If the arteries to the brain become obstructed, there is death of brain tissue because the brain tissue is cut off from sufficient oxygen and other nutrients to continue its normal metabolism and function. Atherosclerosis, by building up in the arteries and ultimately blocking them, thus leads to the major causes of death, heart disease and stroke.

There are many theories to explain the development of atherosclerosis, or hardening of the arteries, but regardless of theory, there remains the well-established direct relation between high blood pressure and atherosclerosis. The Framingham, Massachusetts, study begun in 1948, under the auspices of the United States Public Health Service and the direction of Drs. Thomas R. Dawber and William B. Kannel, was one of the first large-scale investigations to point out the importance of high blood pressure and other factors in the development of atherosclerosis. Permission was obtained from the would-be participants, local doctors, and citizen groups to enlist the cooperation of the population of Framingham. Once this cooperation was assured, a complete medical history was taken and a physical examination performed on each consenting individual. Anyone suffering from heart disease due to atherosclerosis was excluded from the study. Atherosclerotic heart diseases include, for example, heart attacks, also called coronaries and myocardial infarctions. The remaining population, which was free from such disease, was then subjected to a battery of tests: their blood pressure was measured; their height, weight, smoking, and eating habits determined; their family histories recorded; and many blood and urine tests obtained.

They were then told to live their normal lives but were reminded to return every two years for repeated examinations. The expected happened. With the passage of time some of the people who were initially free of atherosclerotic heart disease developed it, and, over time, the numbers increased.

Comparisons could then be made between those who developed this heart disease and those who did not. What led to the increased risk of developing atherosclerotic heart disease? Several factors appeared over and over again: a family history of the disease, a history of smoking, obesity, and perhaps most importantly, increased blood pressure and higher concentrations of cholesterol in the blood. The natural question: what could you do if you had one or more of these risk factors?

The Cholesterol Question

Cholesterol, a fat, is an often-mentioned risk factor in nonmedical discussions on the prevention of atherosclerotic heart disease. It is one of the many food substances the cells need to metabolize in order to maintain life. Normal limits have been defined for cholesterol in much the same way as for blood pressure. When the cholesterol in your blood exceeds that of most of the population you are considered to have "high cholesterol." Evidence shows the lower your cholesterol, the lower the risk of developing atherosclerosis. Similarly, as the amount of cholesterol increases, the risk of developing atherosclerosis is also greater.

It is a normal process for cholesterol to move in and out of arteries. This food substance is filtered through and supplies nutrients to the artery itself. With high cholesterol levels, there tends to be more movement in than out of the arteries. Since atherosclerosis is in part the deposition of fat and blood clots within the arteries, and cholesterol is one of these fats, the ground is laid for the development of atherosclerosis.

High blood pressure compounds the risk. Working together with high levels of cholesterol, higher blood pressure within the vessel forces more cholesterol into the artery wall. If you have high cholesterol but a low blood pressure, the risk of atherosclerosis is relatively reduced. Since cholesterol levels and blood pressure, unlike genetic characteristics, can be partly altered, much effort to combat atherosclerosis has been directed toward reducing levels of this fatty food substance.

Diet has become important. For example, one should avoid foods such as eggs, because the yolk has exceedingly high cholesterol; fatty steaks, which contain saturated animal fats, help raise cholesterol. Butter and rich desserts also have relatively high cholesterol levels or too much saturated fat. Polyunsaturated fats, usually vegetable fats, have been substituted in our diets to reduce our intake of saturated fats. Soft margarine is one example. It has been assumed that if you can lower cholesterol by changing your diet, you can lower the risk of hardening of the arteries and coronary disease and stroke.

The rationale is sound and supported by many investigations. Numerous studies on the origins of atherosclerosis have shown that populations with high cholesterol have more hardening of the arteries and atherosclerotic heart disease than populations with low cholesterol, and this phenomenon has been linked to diet. But in reality, blood cholesterol level is not determined solely by diet. In much the same way that you may inherit a tendency toward high blood pressure, you may also inherit a tendency for high or low cholesterol. If your baseline cholesterol level is high, even if you strictly adhere to a rigorous and controlled diet, you will still end up with relatively high cholesterol compared to the rest of the population. The importance of dietary measures in the control of high cholesterol in the blood is still an area of medical controversy, and the results of some studies have cast a shadow on diet enthusiasts.

A recent United States Veterans Administration investigation is one such study. It took two groups of veterans, and gave one group of men a normal, fatty American diet and the other a low-cholesterol diet that substituted polyunsaturated fats for the saturated fats found in fatty meats and dairy products. After five years the two groups were examined to see whether there was a difference in the development of atherosclerotic heart disease.

The investigators indeed found a difference between the two groups, and in the expected direction. There were fewer complications of atherosclerotic disease, such as heart attacks and strokes, in the group eating a low-fat diet. However, the death rate from all causes was higher within the group with a lower-fat diet than in the group that indulged in the richer, fattier foods. Were the results due to chance? We do not yet know.

With the development of new medical drugs, other modes of treatment are used that can lower cholesterol by impeding the biochemical buildup of this fatty food substance within the blood. These drugs act effectively, and there is good evidence that they may protect people who have high blood cholesterol levels. Since there is evidence that cholesterol may be lowered in the range of 10 to 15 percent by such drugs, they may significantly lessen the risk of developing atherosclerosis. But if your cholesterol is relatively normal, the possible ill effects caused by such drugs might well exceed any benefits.

At the present time we simply do not know the best possible balance between diet and prevention of atherosclerosis. In the meantime, the golden mean of moderation might serve until results are more conclusive. There is little doubt your diet should be modified to lower your blood cholesterol if the level is high. However, this does not mean that people who consume normal amounts of cholesterol should modify their diet. Many physicians feel that if diet is indeed to be changed to include less fat and to be effective, the alteration should occur early and be a lifelong habit.

A Disease With No Symptoms

Let's return to high blood pressure, or hypertension. High blood pressure may be dangerous. Not only does it increase development of atherosclerosis, but high blood pressure itself may cause vessels to burst. It also requires the heart to pump blood at higher pressures, thus making the heart work harder. Pumping at higher pressures places an excessive strain on the heart and the heart grows larger, as would any muscle that is worked excessively. A weight lifter's muscles increase in size because he does the work of lifting barbells. So will heart muscle increase in size or bulk when doing the work of pumping harder. This results in what is called hypertensive heart disease, in which the heart is enlarged (see Figure 6).

Ordinarily, no symptoms are associated with high blood pressure for many years. You simply have the measurable finding of high blood pressure. The insidiousness of hypertension lies in its covert, seemingly harmless nature, which can end in permanent damage to the heart or brain or, at worst, in sudden death. Death of heart or brain tissue occurs either directly, through bursting vessels or an enlarging heart, or indirectly, through the development of atherosclerosis.

When atherosclerosis does develop, when high blood pressure actually brings about hardening of the arteries, the target is usually one or more of three organ systems: the heart, the brain, or the kidneys. The heart is the work organ. As previously noted, it must generate the increased blood pressure by pumping more forcefully and as a result the muscle fibers within the heart increase in size, enlarging the heart. The slow but steady process turns into a vicious cycle: as the heart enlarges to pump, it requires more blood flow through its own coronary arteries to maintain its own increased requirements. The enlarged heart is then more prone to have a heart attack, where heart muscle cells die because the nutrient demands of the heart are not met. Why did it not get sufficient nutrients? At the same time that the heart, because of high blood pressure, enlarges and needs more blood flow to bring nutrients, the coronary arteries become progressively less able to carry larger quantities of blood, because of their inability to enlarge and also because of the increased development of atherosclerosis within these arteries.

High blood pressure affects the brain either directly, through high pressure that leads to bursting of blood vessels, a brain hemorrhage (see Figure 6), or indirectly, through the blockage of arteries by atherosclerosis. These events lead to temporary or permanent damage of brain functions called stroke or shock.

The third set of organs affected is the kidneys. Because of their normal role in blood pressure control, when they become diseased by high blood pressure, they make the high blood pressure worse. In the normal kidney, if blood pressure decreases to very low levels the kidneys secrete hormone substances that increase blood pressure. The kidneys therefore act as sensors to maintain adequate blood pressure. If a minimal amount of atherosclerosis develops in the blood vessels of the kidneys, it will decrease the amount of blood flow to these organs, and the kidneys will become shrunken (see Figure 6). The blocked kidney vessel leads to lower pressure within the kidney, and this organ responds in turn by secreting hormones that raise blood pressure throughout the body. We have a vicious cycle. The raising of

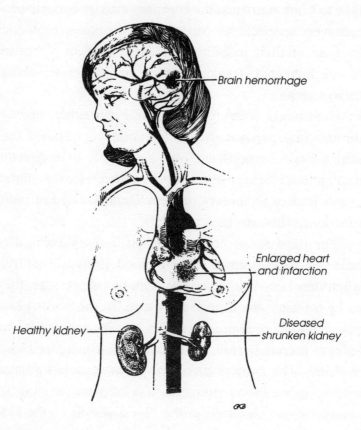

Figure 6
Diagram showing a subject with a large heart from high blood pressure.
The subject's heart has also had an infarction (a heart attack). In this
diagram, other consequences of high blood pressure are pictured: a brain
hemorrhage and a diseased, shrunken kidney.

blood pressure actually leads to the development of more atherosclerosis; blood flow to the kidneys is further blocked by atherosclerosis, which leads to even higher blood pressure.

The solution is to stop the cycle before it begins. There is no mystique in the often repeated formula: the higher your blood pressure, the more likely you are to develop certain heart diseases, strokes, and kidney ailments. Science has not yet discovered why some people and not others are prone to have high blood pressure, or hypertension.

Hypertension is insidiously symptomless throughout its course. Though high blood pressure in some people may not have reached the point where it has become apparent by causing the diseases associated with it, doctors today are more apt to consider the physical findings of high blood pressure itself to be a disease state. Arbitrary limits have been drawn to dictate what is high blood pressure, what is normal, and what is in between high and normal, called borderline high blood pressure. High blood pressure is arbitrarily considered to be pressure greater than 159 millimeters of mercury* systolic or 94 diastolic. Borderline high blood pressure is considered to be either between 140 and 159 systolic or between 90

---

*Blood pressure is expressed in terms of millimeters of mercury. A column of mercury is raised a specific number of millimeters by a specific pressure. The higher the pressure, the higher the column is raised.

and 94 diastolic. Normal blood pressure is defined as lower than 140 systolic and 90 diastolic.*

At this point in medical knowledge we can identify the cause of only approximately 5 to 10 percent of the cases of high blood pressure; for 90 to 95 percent of the cases of hypertension we cannot. We know the cause when some of the body's mechanisms that control blood pressure are not functioning properly. As noted, the kidneys secrete potent substances within the bloodstream that will raise blood pressure, when they sense a lower blood pressure.

Indeed, one of the first ways hypertension was produced in animals was through experiments performed in the nineteen-thirties by Dr. H. Goldblatt, who discovered the relation between the kidneys and the elevation of blood pressure. In dogs, after removing one of the two kidneys, he placed a clamp on the artery leading to the other. He thus decreased the blood pressure of the remaining kidney. Secretion of kidney hormones followed, which resulted in permanent hypertension, or high blood pressure, in the dogs. From that time on, much of the search for the cause of hypertension was drawn to malfunctions of the kidney. Certainly, in about 2 to 5 percent of cases of hypertension the cause may be found in a constricted artery going to the kidney. By removing the obstruction, we can cure the hypertension. But this ac-

---

*See Figure 5, page 23 for explanation of systolic and diastolic.

counts for only a very small fraction of the millions of cases of hypertension seen in the United States today.

Very high blood pressure is also sometimes experienced during pregnancy, and this kind of hypertension can be cured. It can be controlled up to the time of delivery. When the mother delivers the baby, her blood pressure most often returns to normal levels. Tumors in the adrenal glands or in the brain can cause high blood pressure and are sometimes curable. Forms of hypertension linked to the thyroid gland can also be cured. Surgery is often used to treat most of these types of hypertension.

But we still do not have an answer for 90 to 95 percent of the cases of hypertension called "essential hypertension." Essential hypertension is hypertension of unknown cause. "Stress" is a generally accepted explanation of hypertension, but there is skepticism among physicians about the role of stress. They are justifiably wary of such a cause-and-effect relation.

What is stress? How do you measure and quantify it? How is stress related to blood pressure? Because of the difficulties of measuring stress, relatively little research has been done on stress and high blood pressure. The reason is similar to the drunk's reason for looking for his cufflink at night under a lighted lamppost, when in fact he had lost the cufflink up the street. Asked why, he replied: "Because the light is better here." The kidneys are organs that have been well investigated, but stress, because of the difficulty of measuring it, has not been studied well. Until recently the light in the above analogy was where the kidneys were; stress was with the cufflink. Though it is commonly assumed that people's feelings such as anger, fear, or anxiety play an important role in causing hypertension, our tools for gathering data in this area have been limited. Consequently, the subject has been inadequately studied. Yet situations leading to continuous behavioral adjustment, perhaps a better way to define what is stressful, may underlie the development of many of the causes of essential hypertension, the 90 to 95 percent of cases of high blood pressure which cannot be explained.

3
.

Stress has long been the subject of psychological and physiologic speculation. In fact, more often than not, the word itself is ill-defined and overused, meaning different things to different people. Emotional stress, for example, can come about as the result of a family argument or the death of a loved one. Environmental stress, such as exposure to excessive heat or cold, is an entirely different phenomenon. Physiologic stress has been described as the outpouring of the steroid hormones from the adrenal glands, a theory elaborated upon by Dr. Hans Selye of Montreal, who believes these hormones are vitally important for the survival of an organism and are exquisitely sensitive indices of stress. Whatever its guise, a lack of a firm definition has seriously impeded past research.

Drs. Thomas H. Holmes and Richard H. Rahe, psychiatrists at the University of Washington Medical School, have devised a scale of stressful events. Hundreds of persons of varying ages, backgrounds, and classes were asked to rank the relative amount of adjustment required to meet a series of life events. Holmes and Rahe have called this list "the social readjustment scale." The scale is based on interviews with 394 individuals. The actual numerical rating was the average number of units these individuals assigned to the various life events after being told marriage was equivalent to fifty units. Heading the list is death of a spouse. The doctors subsequently found that ten times more widows and widowers die during the first year after the death of their husbands or wives than all others in their age group; that divorced persons have an illness rate twelve times higher than married persons in the year following the divorce. According to the doctors, change, whether for "good" or "bad," causes stress to a human being, leaving him more susceptible to disease.

TABLE 1
THE STRESS OF ADJUSTING TO CHANGE

Events	*Scale of Impact*
Death of spouse	100
Divorce	73
Marital separation	65
Jail term	63
Death of close family member	63
Personal injury or illness	53
Marriage	50
Fired at work	47
Marital reconciliation	45
Retirement	45
Change in health of family member	44
Pregnancy	40
Sex difficulties	39
Gain of new family member	39
Business readjustment	39
Change in financial state	38
Death of close friend	37
Change to different line of work	36
Change in number of arguments with spouse	35
Mortgage over $10,000	31
Foreclosure of mortgage or loan	30

Events	Scale of Impact
Change in responsibilities at work	29
Son or daughter leaving home	29
Trouble with in-laws	29
Outstanding personal achievement	28
Wife begins or stops work	26
Begin or end school	26
Change in living conditions	25
Revision of personal habits	24
Trouble with boss	23
Change in work hours or conditions	20
Change in residence	20
Change in schools	20
Change in recreation	19
Change in church activities	19
Change in social activities	18
Mortgage or loan less than $10,000	17
Change in sleeping habits	16
Change in number of family get-togethers	15
Change in eating habits	15
Vacation	13
Christmas	12
Minor violations of the law	11

Our approach is similar in that we define stress as environmental conditions that require *behavioral adjustment*. For example, stressful circumstances are those associated with rapid cultural change, urbanization and migration, socioeconomic mobility, or uncertainty in the immediate environment. I formulated this working definition in the course of early studies in collaboration with Dr. Mary C. Gutmann at the Harvard Medical School's Thorndike Memorial and Channing Laboratories at the Boston City Hospital. The research provided a starting point for measuring how stress interacts with blood pressure.

Who Develops Hypertension?

Life-threatening events are the most obvious environmental circumstances requiring behavioral adjustment. On April 16, 1947, a ship containing explosive material blew up in Texas City with a blast estimated to equal the force of the Bikini atomic bombs. Practicing physicians in the area, according to a study, found a marked increase in the blood pressures of their patients for days after the explosion. During World War II, physicians observed elevated blood pressures among the besieged Russian population of Leningrad, as they did among soldiers going to battle.

Less dramatic but more immediately relevant is what happens to people who have to adjust to city living. Several studies have examined how individuals are affected when social roles break down and they are forced to establish new ones. Tests have shown that high blood pressure goes hand in hand with adjustment to city life. For example, one of our studies demonstrated that citizens living in Puerto Rican rural areas had practically no hypertension. In contrast, 18 percent of their counterparts living within a Puerto Rican metropolitan area had blood pressures in the hypertensive range. Higher blood pressure paralleled the degree of "Westernization" of Fiji Islanders. Members of an African Zulu tribe also showed a rise in blood pressure after migration from primitive to urban areas. Stress associated with the adjustment of becoming a city dweller is felt to be an important contributory factor in hypertension. Consider the high rate of job mobility in our society and the frequency of families being uprooted. During a lifetime Americans may move from one to ten times or more, whether from a rural to an urban environment or from one city to another. We can now begin to appreciate how frequently behavioral adjustment is demanded of us in our open society.

More than geographical change and social readjustment may be involved in moving up the so-called occupational ladder. Reaching a long-sought-after, desirable position, for which you do not feel adequately prepared, can raise blood pressure. Drs. L. E. Hinkle and H. G.

Wolff measured the blood pressure of college and high-school graduates who moved into "white-collar" jobs and found the less educated had higher blood pressures. The white-collar job required greater behavioral adjustment for those with less education than for the college graduates.

Other studies bear out the close relation between the environment and hypertension and at the same time question the accepted view that blacks are genetically more susceptible to high blood pressure than whites. Recently, a widely distributed health pamphlet issued by the Health Insurance Plan of Greater New York offered the following information: "High blood pressure is the principal disease suffered by blacks in this country, and an important factor contributing to their shorter life-expectancy. The number of blacks in young-adulthood and middle age suffering from the disease ranges from three to twelve times higher than that of whites. More seem to develop it earlier in life and there are more fatalities at a younger age."

Is the reason a genetic factor or is it the need for behavioral adjustment? Dr. E. Harburg and associates at the University of Michigan found that blacks tested in "high stress" neighborhoods of Detroit were more likely to have high blood pressure than blacks in middle-class neighborhoods. The black people who felt forever trapped within the ghetto had very high blood pressures. Certainly, ghetto life requires continuous behavioral adjustment.

In Mississippi, where white and black high-school women were matched for socioeconomic status, measurements revealed that there were no differences in level of blood pressure. When you compared whites with blacks when both had the same standard of living, the blood pressures of the whites were as high as the blacks'. These results thus seriously question the long-held view of disproportionate black susceptibility to high blood pressure. The degree of high blood pressure among blacks is not simply genetic but probably is related to the living standards and stress under which black people exist.

Whether it be urban-rural differences or ghetto existence, the need for behavioral adjustment is there, and this need may well underlie the amount of high blood pressure observed today. We live in very difficult times, when man is constantly faced with anxieties caused by rapid change. Man simply does not have the biological resources to maintain physiologic equanimity, certainly not without experiencing the effects of so-called stress that may have led to the recent marked prevalence of the disease hypertension. As A. M. Osfeld and R. B. Shekelle, of the University of Illinois College of Medicine, put it, "There has been an appreciable increase in uncertainty of human relations as man has gone from the relatively primitive and more rural to the urban and industrial. Contemporary man, in much of the world, is faced every day with people and with situations about which there is uncertainty of outcome, wherein appropriate behavior is not prescribed and validated by tradition, where the possibility of bodily or psychological harm exists, where running or fighting is inappropriate, and where mental vigilance is called for." The elevation of blood pressure will depend upon the extent to which the individual is exposed to accelerated environmental change and uncertainty, and on his innate and acquired abilities to adapt.

Controversies about the effects of stress have centered not only on issues relating to its ambiguous definition and its psychological and physiologic manifestations but also on how stress affects different individuals. A theory has been proposed that a certain personality type may be more prone to the effects of stress and thus to hypertension—in short, that there may be a hypertensive personality. Is a nervous, anxious individual actually more prone to hypertension than a seemingly calm person? We believe that there is no such thing as a hypertensive personality. Anyone faced often enough with circumstances that require behavioral adjustment can develop hypertension.

The concept of a hypertensive personality evolved from retrospective studies. A retrospective study does the following: it takes a group of people suffering from a disease such as hypertension and measures a variable such as personality trait and then compares the personality traits with those found in a matched group of people who do not suffer from hypertension. Retrospective studies have repeatedly shown that hypertensive individuals are persons who do not deal with their emotions well or who cannot let out their emotions. It was concluded that the subjects suffering from hypertension had a hypertensive personality.

The fallacy of this type of reasoning is obvious, because the disease of hypertension itself may influence personality traits. What is needed are "prospective" studies in which a group of subjects without hypertension should be examined; their personality types should be determined, and they should then be followed over time. Some will probably develop hypertension. When sufficient numbers of subjects have developed the disease, comparisons of the originally noted personality types can be made. No such studies exist.

We reiterate that a crucial factor in the development of high blood pressure is the necessity to cope with an environment requiring continuous behavioral adjustment. Certainly if the environment is as difficult as ours is today, we have to become more aware of the situations that require behavioral adjustment and in turn raise our blood pressure. This is a new direction in how we should think about stress. We can either change the complexities of life—an unlikely event, for they are likely to increase—or develop ways that enable us to cope more effectively.

Internal Signs of Stress

Much has been said up to now about situations that require behavioral adjustment and their relation to high blood pressure. But what happens physiologically? By what mechanisms do these situations requiring behavioral adjustment lead to high blood pressure? Man instinctively reacts to such situations by unconsciously activating the fight-or-flight response.

This fight-or-flight response was first described by Dr. Walter B. Cannon, a celebrated professor of physiology at the Harvard Medical School at the turn of the twentieth century, as an "emergency reaction." As we discussed in Chapter 1, the response prepares the animal for running or fighting. Changes include increased blood pressure; increased heart rate; increased rate of breathing; increased body metabolism, or rate of burning fuel; and marked increase in the flow of blood to the muscles of the arms and legs (see Figure 7). We believe the more often the fight-or-flight response is activated, the more likely it is that you will develop high blood pressure, especially if circumstances do not allow you to actually give battle or flee.

A Czech scientist, Dr. J. Brod, and his associates substantiated the physiologic characteristics of the response in a classic experiment in which he took a group of healthy, young, normal adults and measured blood pressure, as well as all the blood pumped by the heart, and the specific amount pumped to the muscles. For baseline measures, he had the participants lie quietly while he took measurements of these internal functions. He then gave them an arithmetic problem to solve: from a four-digit number like 1,194, subtract consecutive serial 17's. He said "Go" and had them subtract 17 from the first number and 17 from the answer, down the line, to the background beat of a metronome going click, click, click. He also gathered friends around them making statements like "I did better than that." Click, click.

You can guess what happened: increased blood pressure, increased muscle blood flow, increased pumping of blood by the heart, showing that this same integrated fight-or-flight response is not only still with us but could occur in response to the very simple psychological challenge of mental arithmetic under time pressure. Multiply these measured reactions by what happens to most of us in the course of our daily lives and it is obvious how the fight-or-flight response can cause transient high blood pressure. Now you can see how situations that require behavioral adjustment can lead to specific physiologic changes, which bring forth the fight-or-flight response. We are all basically the same human organism, which responds to stressful events through this common, innate response. We may differ in what is stressful to us individually, depending upon our own value systems, but our society poses enough stressful circumstances to affect all of us.

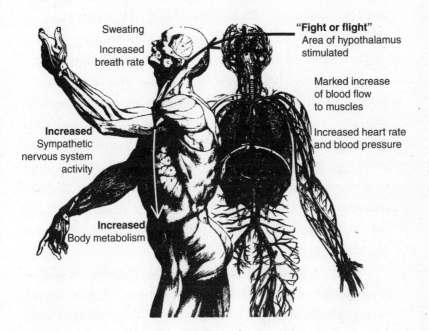

Figure 7
Physiologic changes associated with the fight-or-flight response. (Sixteenth-century anatomical drawing by Vesalius.)

Further research demonstrates that the chronic elicitation of the fight-or-flight response leads from the transient elevations in blood pressure to a permanent state of hypertension. Drs. B. Folkow and E. H. Rubinstein, at the University of Göteborg in Sweden, implanted wires in the brains of rats in an area called the hypothalamus (see Figure 8). It is the hypothalamus that controls the evocation of the fight-or-flight response. The response could be evoked when the researchers passed an electric current through the wire. They then divided these rats into two groups, but stimulated the electrodes in only one group. Higher blood pressure developed in the rats stimulated to activate the fight-or-flight response. Those rats not subject to electrical stimulation maintained lower blood pressures.

When a single situation requiring behavioral adjustment occurs again and again, the fight-or-flight response is repeatedly activated. Ultimately, this repetition may lead to higher blood pressure on a permanent basis. It is our underlying theory that this is what happens in man in the development of permanent hypertension. The chronic arousal of the fight-or-flight response goes from the just transient elevation in blood pressure to permanent high blood pressure.

In the past, the fight-or-flight response had considerable evolutionary significance. Individuals with this response could survive more effectively, passing it on to their offspring. Though we chronically evoke the re-

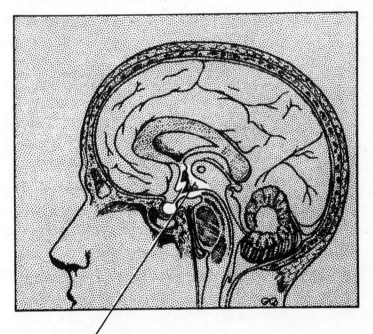

Hypothalamic area

Figure 8
The hypothalamic area of the brain.

sponse, modern society does not socially accept the fighting or running naturally associated with it. For example, you obviously do not run away from or hit your boss when he or she yells at you. Our innate reactions have not changed, but society has. The response is turned on, but we do not use it appropriately.

When the fight-or-flight response is evoked, a part of the *involuntary* nervous system called the sympathetic nervous system becomes highly active. If you want to lift your arm, you can willfully control the skeletal musculature of the *voluntary* nervous system to do so. The involuntary, or autonomic, nervous system deals with the everyday bodily functions that normally do not come into consciousness, such as the maintenance of heartbeat and blood pressure, regular breathing, the digestion of food. When the fight-or-flight response is evoked, it brings into play the sympathetic nervous system, which is part of the autonomic, or involuntary, nervous system. The sympathetic nervous system acts by secreting specific hormones: adrenalin or epinephrine and noradrenalin or norepinephrine. These hormones, epinephrine and its related substances, bring about the physiologic changes of increased blood pressure, heart rate, and body metabolism.

The fight-or-flight response happens in an integrated fashion. It is integrated because it is controlled by a part of an area in the brain called the hypothalamus (see Figure 8) and most, if not all, of the response occurs in a coordinated, simultaneous manner. Electrically stimulate a specific area of the hypothalamus and there will be an outpouring of adrenalin or epinephrine and related hormones controlled by the sympathetic nervous system with the associated physiologic changes.

While the fight-or-flight response is associated with the overactivity of the sympathetic nervous system, there is another response that leads to a quieting of the same nervous system. Indeed, there is evidence that hypertensive subjects can lower their blood pressure by regularly eliciting this other response. This is the Relaxation Response, an opposite, involuntary response that causes a reduction in the activity of the sympathetic nervous system (see Figure 9, page 54). Since we cannot easily change the nature of modern life, perhaps better prevention and therapy of hypertension and other diseases related to the fight-or-flight response might be achieved by actively bringing forth the Relaxation Response.

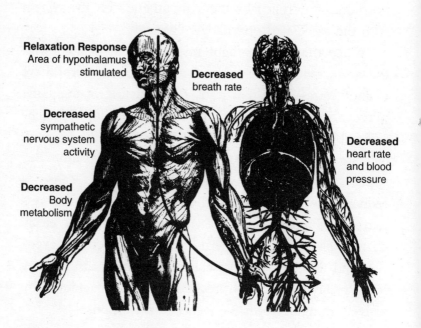

Relaxation Response
Area of hypothalamus stimulated

Decreased breath rate

Decreased sympathetic nervous system activity

Decreased heart rate and blood pressure

Decreased Body metabolism

Figure 9
Physiologic changes associated with the Relaxation Response. (Sixteenth-century anatomical drawing by Vesalius.)

4

·

Are we really able to adjust to physiologically jarring changes in our environment? We are being tested today more rigorously than ever before. As we saw in Chapter 3, the repeated and inappropriate arousal of the fight-or-flight response suggests that we may not be capable of adapting ourselves either psychologically or physiologically as fast as the environment around us changes. Indeed, the prevalence of hypertension and the rapid rise of deaths from heart disease and stroke strongly suggest that we are not. Since the environment is unlikely to grow less complex or more stable, we must find within our own bodies a physiologic means of dealing with the demands of twenty-first-century life. Can we influence our own physiologic reaction to stress through individually controlled mental practices?

Mental Control

Behavioral experiments have addressed this problem for several decades. Dr. B. F. Skinner, of Harvard University, showed the extent to which behavior is determined by environment. *Alter the environment and you can control behavior.* Skinner's behavioral experiments dealt with *overt skeletal muscular* effects, such as training an animal to press a key or lever in the presence of what he called the reinforcer, a reward that would increase the likelihood that the animal would do it again. For example, if he wanted a pigeon to peck at a certain key, each time the pigeon moved closer to that key Skinner would reward it with a pellet of food. When it moved even closer, another pellet would be there as a reward. Eventually, by guiding and shaping the animal through reinforcement, the pellet of food, Skinner trained the pigeon to peck time and again at the desired key. Skinner thus succeeded in "shaping" the voluntary muscular behavior of the animal.

Dr. Neil E. Miller took Skinner's research a significant

step further into the autonomic nervous system, saying that one can alter not only voluntary muscular behavior but also a subject's involuntary behavior. Through Miller's work, control of involuntary bodily processes was shown to be possible through *biofeedback*. A forerunner in the field, Miller showed through years of experimentation that involuntary bodily processes, such as the amount of blood flowing to an animal's ear, could be changed.

Experiments centering on biofeedback involve rewarding desired performance, which in turn alters internal bodily functions. In brief, then, proponents of biofeedback believe that by mentally recognizing a biologic function you can gain control of that function. We have long been aware that man's skeletal muscles are commanded by his voluntary nerves acting through the brain. However, Western man has only recently recognized that he can control his involuntary responses. The regulator of these involuntary processes such as blood pressure, heartbeat, and amount of blood flow to various parts of the body is called the autonomic nervous system. Visceral learning, or biofeedback, as it is popularly called, established that man could control his involuntary or autonomic nervous system.

Using the concepts of biofeedback, Miller trained rats to alter a number of internal involuntary acts by appropriate rewards and punishments. He accomplished this by monitoring the rats' physiologic functions following certain changes and then signaling, or feeding back, rewards for changes in the desired direction. The "biofeedback" of Miller is based upon the "operant conditioning" of Skinner. Miller's methods of rewards and punishment paralleled Skinner's reinforcements, and in this way he was able to shape autonomic, or so-called involuntary, functions.

We have used operant conditioning and biofeedback to demonstrate the behavioral control of blood pressure.* Devising a system that would "feed back" information about blood pressure levels to a group of laboratory monkeys, we trained these monkeys to raise or lower their blood pressures through the use of rewards and punishments. We have also shown that hypertensive *human beings* were capable of lowering their blood pressure. Before we started these investigations we obtained the approval of both a Harvard and a Boston City Hospital Human Studies Committee whose purpose is to protect the rights and safety of volunteers in any scientific study. Before each study, the subjects' rights and risks were thoroughly explained and each gave his written informed consent. In this investigation, we attached the patients to monitors that kept them informed of momentary rises or falls of blood pressure. Through the use of such feedback, our

---

*Collaborators in the research involving monkeys were Drs. J. A. Herd, W. H. Morse, R. T. Kelleher, A. C. Barger, and P. B. Dews. Drs. D. Shapiro, B. Tursky, and G. E. Schwartz were collaborators in the human investigations.

patients apparently learned to lower their systolic blood pressure levels. But when we asked these subjects how they lowered their blood pressures, they said simply that they did so by thinking relaxing thoughts. If that was so, we reasoned, why should we bother with the biofeedback apparatus?

After all, biofeedback has several major drawbacks. Usually no more than one physiologic function at a time can be fed back upon and thus changed. Also, biofeedback involves a great deal of costly equipment; the physiologic changes that are going on must be carefully monitored. Heart rate, for example, must be monitored and measured on a beat-to-beat basis, so you can recognize when heart rate goes up or down, and reward in the appropriate direction. Although Miller demonstrated experimentally that involuntary functions could be purposefully altered, subsequent systematic research showed us that the same result could be achieved by methods other than biofeedback.

But centuries before such research, dramatic claims for control of physiologic functions had already come to us from the East. According to these claims, physiologic functions could be controlled through the use of the ancient meditational techniques of Yoga and Zen Buddhism. Yoga, a part of Indian culture for thousands of years, is the culmination of ancient Hindu efforts to give man the fullest possible control over his mind. In New Delhi, Dr. B. K. Anand and two collaborators studied a

Yogi who had been confined in a sealed metal box. They reported he was able to slow his oxygen consumption, or metabolism, an involuntary mechanism partly related to the sympathetic nervous system. Claims have been made of more phenomenal feats, such as voluntarily stopping the heartbeat. But these claims appear to be based on misinter-pretations of data and are simply erroneous, as is shown in other studies by Drs. B. K. Anand, W. A. Wenger, and B. K. Bagchi. Other researchers in the nineteen-fifties and sixties showed that Zen monks in Japan highly expe-rienced in the practice of deep meditation could also de-crease their oxygen consumption, or metabolism, by as much as 20 percent, a level reached usually only after four or five hours of sleep. These findings indicate that through the control of certain mental, voluntary acts, "in-voluntary" mechanisms in the body, or mechanisms of the autonomic nervous system, can be altered.

Explorations using the electroencephalogram have further confirmed that Yogic and meditational practices produce changes in the electrical activity of the brain. The electroencephalogram is a device that employs wires placed on the scalp and forehead to measure this electri-cal activity. Drs. A. Kasamatsu and T. Hirai of the Uni-versity of Tokyo discovered that Zen monks who meditated with their eyes half open developed a predomi-nance of alpha waves, brain waves usually associated with feelings of well-being. Furthermore, the alpha waves in-crease in amplitude and regularity during meditation.

B. K. Anand and other investigators in India reported the same heightening of alpha activity during the meditation of Yogis.

Yoga, Zen, and other forms of meditation have found their way into Western life. Transcendental Meditation, one of the most widely practiced forms of meditation, first gained popularity in the nineteen-sixties, when it attracted the Beatles, Mia Farrow, and other celebrities. T.M., as it is also called, now claims worldwide practitioners numbering between five hundred thousand and two million people.

In 1968, practitioners of Transcendental Meditation came to the laboratory at the Harvard Medical School, where we were in the midst of studying the relation between a monkey's behavior and his blood pressure. These devotees of meditation asked whether they could be studied, for they felt they could lower their blood pressure through Transcendental Meditation. They were turned away with a polite "Thank you." Why investigate anything so far out as meditation?

However, these practitioners of Transcendental Meditation were not daunted by this first turndown. They persisted, and the initial No became a Yes. I felt there was little to lose in a preliminary investigation and the potential gains were great. Studies to determine whether meditation could lower blood pressure were then launched. This research at Harvard was conducted independently of other investigations then under way in California. The

California studies were being made by R. Keith Wallace, a Ph.D. candidate in physiology at the University of California, Los Angeles, working closely with Dr. Archie K. Wilson. After obtaining his doctorate based upon physiologic studies in T.M., Dr. Wallace joined the research team at Harvard's Thorndike Memorial Laboratory of the Boston City Hospital.

As a first step, known studies on meditators were carefully reviewed, yielding a bewildering range of cases and results. We found that subjects, particularly practitioners of various forms of Yoga, varied greatly in meditative techniques, expertise, and performance. All sought a "higher" consciousness but in different ways: some through a fully rested, relaxed body and a fully awake, relaxed mind; some through strenuous physical exercise; and still others by concentrating on controlling certain functions such as breathing. The need for rigorous discipline and long training allowed for even greater variability in results. Who were the experts and how could we assess their expertise? Fortunately, from a scientific standpoint, Transcendental Meditation, developed by Maharishi Mahesh Yogi, is a simple Yogic technique carried out under reasonably uniform conditions.

A great debt is owed Maharishi Mahesh Yogi, a guru, who early in his life had studied physics. Following the teachings of his mentor, Shri Guru Deva, he eliminated from Yoga certain elements that he considered to be nonessential. He left India, bringing with him this revised form of Yoga which could be grasped more easily by Westerners. He then set up an organization to train instructors who in turn could teach his technique. His methods do not require intense concentration or any form of rigorous mental or physical control. As a result, practically all initiates can easily "meditate" after a short training course.

Transcendental Meditation involves a surprisingly simple technique. A trained instructor gives you a secret word or sound or phrase, a mantra, which you promise not to divulge. This sound is allegedly chosen to suit the individual and is to be silently "perceived." The meditator receives the mantra from his teacher and then repeats it mentally over and over again while sitting in a comfortable position. The purpose of this repetition is to prevent distracting thoughts. Meditators are told to assume a passive attitude and if other thoughts come into mind to disregard them, going back to the mantra. Practitioners are advised to meditate twenty minutes in the morning, usually before breakfast, and twenty minutes in the evening, usually before dinner. We used the technique of the Maharishi Mahesh Yogi as a meditation-Yoga model to help us understand the effects of meditation on blood pressure and other physiologic functions.

Before beginning the tests, I met with the Maharishi to establish whether he would be willing to cooperate with the new research even if the findings proved to be detrimental to his movement. Convinced that only beneficial results would follow, the Maharishi readily agreed to accept any research findings. Once the decision was made to study the meditators, there was no problem getting volunteers, since Maharishi's followers strongly felt what they were doing was beneficial to themselves and mankind. Furthermore, at the time, there was no published material on what happened during the practice of Transcendental Meditation. Approval by Harvard Human Studies Committees was again obtained and written informed consent was given by the subjects.

Volunteers included several who were working for the Transcendental Meditation society. Others were full-time students, mathematicians, artists, and businessmen. Their ages ranged from seventeen to forty-one years, and the length of time they had practiced meditation extended from less than a month to over nine years. A majority had been practicing meditation for two to three years. Each participant in the study was seated in a chair, measuring devices were attached or inserted, and a thirty-minute period allowed so that the subject could adjust to the instruments. Then, measurements were started and continued for three periods: twenty to thirty minutes of sitting quietly, twenty to thirty minutes of practicing meditation, and another twenty to thirty minutes of sitting quietly after the subject was told to stop meditating.

Sleep vs. Meditation

The experiments showed that during meditation there was a *marked decrease in the body's oxygen consumption* (see Figure 10). As mentioned in Chapter 2, each cell makes use of the energy in foods by slowly "burning" the nutrients. In order to "burn" the nutrients the cell usually utilizes oxygen brought to it through the bloodstream. The sum of the individual metabolism of each of the cells utilizing oxygen constitutes the total oxygen consumption, or metabolism, of the body. The major physiologic change associated with meditation is a *decrease in the rate of metabolism* (see Figure 9). Such a state of decreased metabolism, called *hypometabolism,* is a restful state. Like sleep, another hypometabolic state, meditation causes bodily energy resources to be taxed less.

Humans rarely achieve a hypometabolic state, associated with an oxygen consumption that is lower than occurs when you sit quietly in a chair or lie down. In fact, there are very few conditions that lead to hypometabolism. Sleep is one; hibernation is another. Since oxygen consumption is significantly lowered during the practice of meditation, it was first thought this decreased consumption of oxygen might be due to an unknown hibernation-like response in people. One way to know whether hibernation is occurring is to measure the body's rectal temperature. During hibernation this temperature decreases. Meditators, it appears, do not hibernate. Their rectal temperatures do not decrease during the practice of meditation.

Are the physiologic changes associated with meditation the same as those found in sleep, another hypometabolic state? There is little resemblance. During both sleep and meditation there is a decrease in oxygen consumption. However, there are marked differences in the rate of oxygen-consumption decrease during sleep and meditation. During sleep, oxygen consumption decreases slowly and progressively, until, after four or five hours, it is about 8 percent lower than during wakefulness. During meditation, however, the decrease averages between 10 and 20 percent and occurs during the first three minutes of meditation (see Figure 11). It is not possible for a person to bring about such decreases by other means. For example, if you hold your breath, your tissues will continue to utilize the available oxygen at the same rate and there will be no change in the amount of oxygen you consume.

Another physiologic difference between meditation and sleep has been documented with the electroencephalogram. Alpha waves, slow brain waves, increase in intensity and frequency during the practice of meditation but are not commonly found in sleep. We still do not know the significance of alpha waves, but, as previously noted, we do know that they are present when people feel relaxed. Other brain-wave patterns during meditation are also distinctly different from those during sleep. For ex-

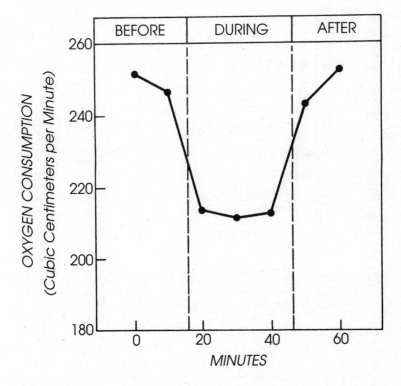

Figure 10
Oxygen-consumption changes associated with the Relaxation Response.
Note the marked decrease in the rate of metabolism.

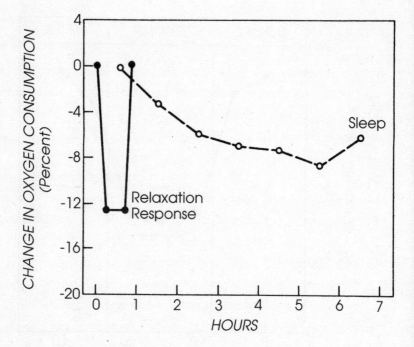

Figure 11
Comparison of the change in oxygen consumption which occurs during the Relaxation Response with that which occurs during sleep. The decreased metabolism during the Relaxation Response continues as long as the response is being elicited.

ample, none or few of the brain-wave electric signals characteristic of rapid eye movement, often seen in sleep and associated with dreaming, are recorded during meditation.

Meditation is therefore not a form of sleep; nor can it be used as a substitute for sleep. Meditation evokes *some* of the physiologic changes that are found in sleep, but the two are not in any way interchangeable, nor is one a substitute for the other. In fact, a look into the sleeping habits of meditators left us with reports that some slept more after regularly practicing meditation and others less. Some noted no change at all.

Along with the drop in oxygen consumption and alpha-wave production during meditation, there is a marked decrease in blood lactate, a substance produced by the metabolism of skeletal muscles and of particular interest because of its purported association with anxiety (see Figure 12). In 1967, Drs. F. N. Pitts, Jr., and J. N. McLure, Jr., of the Washington University School of Medicine, in St. Louis, investigated a group of patients who suffered from neurosis and frequent attacks of anxiety. They injected into their subjects either a nonactive salt solution or a solution of lactate. (The bottles were mixed so that neither the subjects nor the physicians knew which was being infused.) They found that when lactate was being infused, practically every patient with anxiety neurosis experienced an anxiety attack. If the other salt solutions were injected, the percentage of anxi-

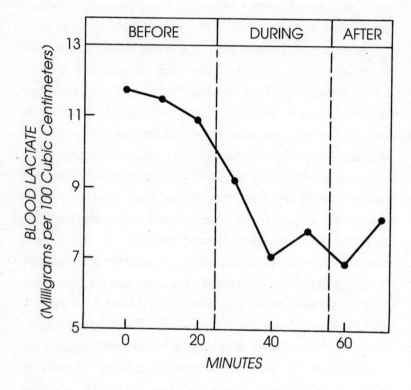

Figure 12
Blood-lactate changes associated with the Relaxation Response.

ety attacks fell significantly. When they took normal people and infused lactate into them, they found that 20 percent of these "normal" people would experience an anxiety attack while practically none would experience an anxiety attack when the nonactive salt solution was injected.

If increased lactate is instrumental in producing regular attacks of anxiety, the finding of low levels of lactate in meditators is consistent with their reports of significantly more relaxed, less anxious feelings. Blood-lactate levels fall rapidly within the first ten minutes of meditation. Though the reason for decreased lactate is uncertain, it is consistent with decreased activity of the sympathetic nervous system. This is the system that is activated during elicitation of the fight-or-flight response.

Putting aside changes in oxygen consumption, brain waves, and lactate levels, other measurements supported the concept of meditation as a highly relaxed condition associated with lowered activity in the sympathetic nervous system. In the tests of the volunteer meditators the heart rate decreased on the average about three beats per minute, and respiration rate, or rate of breathing, also slowed. All these physiologic changes in people who were practicing the simply learned technique of Transcendental Meditation were very similar to feats observed in highly trained experts in Yoga and Zen with fifteen to twenty years of concentrated experience in meditation.

What did not change in these early experiments involving young, healthy subjects was blood pressure. The blood pressure of the meditators was low before, during, and after the experiment. Although blood pressures remained unchanged during the practice of meditation, the low blood pressures of the meditators pointed the way to future experiments. Perhaps they had low blood pressure because of their continued practice of meditation. If this was true, the possibility existed that people with hypertension could lower their blood pressures through such a practice.

As the experiments progressed over several years, the concept developed that the various physiologic changes that accompanied Transcendental Meditation were part of an integrated response opposite to the fight-or-flight response and that *they were in no way unique to Transcendental Meditation.* Indeed, lowered oxygen consumption, heart rate, respiration, and blood lactate are indicative of decreased activity of the sympathetic nervous system and represent a *hypometabolic, or restful, state.* On the other hand, the physiologic changes of the fight-or-flight response are associated with increased sympathetic nervous system activity and represent a *hypermetabolic state.*

Dr. Hess's Crucial Experiments

Dr. Walter R. Hess, the Swiss Nobel Prizewinning physiologist, produced the changes associated with the fight-or-flight response by stimulating a part of the cat's brain within the hypothalamus (see Figure 8). Moreover, by stimulating another area within the hypothalamus, Dr. Hess demonstrated a response whose physiologic changes were similar to those measured during the practice of meditation, that is, a response opposite to the fight-or-flight response. He termed this reaction the trophotropic response and described it as "a protective mechanism against overstress belonging to the trophotropic system and promoting restorative processes." The trophotropic response described by Hess in the cat is, we believe, the Relaxation Response in man. Hence, both of these opposite responses are associated with physiologic changes occurring concomitantly in a coordinated fashion and each appears to be controlled by the hypothalamus. Because the fight-or-flight response and the Relaxation Response are in opposition, one counteracts the effects of the other. This is why we feel the Relaxation Response is of such import, for with its regular use it will offset the harmful effects of the inappropriate elicitation of the fight-or-flight response.

As shown in Table 2, there are several techniques, most of which are used as relaxation therapy, which evoke the same physiologic changes as the Relaxation Re-

TABLE 2

DIFFERENT TECHNIQUES ELICITING THE PHYSIOLOGIC CHANGES OF THE RELAXATION RESPONSE

Physiologic Measurement Technique	Oxygen Consumption	Respiratory Rate
Transcendental Meditation	Decreases	Decreases
Zen and Yoga	Decreases	Decreases
Autogenic Training	Not Measured	Decreases
Progressive Relaxation	Not Measured	Not Measured
Hypnosis With Suggested Deep Relaxation	Decreases	Decreases
Sentic Cycles	Decreases	Decreases

Heart Rate	Alpha Waves	Blood Pressure	Muscle Tension
Decreases	Increases	Decreases★	Not Measured
Decreases	Increases	Decreases★	Not Measured
Decreases	Increases	Inconclusive Results	Decreases
Not Measured	Not Measured	Inconclusive Results	Decreases
Decreases	Not Measured	Inconclusive Results	Not Measured
Decreases	Not Measured	Not Measured	Not Measured

★In patients with elevated blood pressure.

sponse. Some of the techniques included in this table, Autogenic Training; Progressive Relaxation; Hypnosis with Suggested Deep Relaxation; and Sentic Cycles, may be unfamiliar to you and will be briefly explained.

Autogenic Training is a technique of medical therapy based on six mental exercises devised by Dr. H. H. Shultz, a German neurologist. It is to be practiced several times a day until the subject is able to shift voluntarily to a purportedly less stressful state, or the trophotropic state of Hess. The room is quiet, you lie down and close your eyes. Exercise One has you focus on a feeling of heaviness in the limbs; and Exercise Two on the sensation of warmth in the limbs. Exercise Three deals with alleged heart regulation, and Exercise Four with passive concentration on breathing. In Exercise Five, the subject cultivates feelings of coolness in the forehead. Exercises One through Four most effectively elicit the Relaxation Response. The subject's attitude toward the exercise, and this is absolutely essential, must not be intense and compulsive, but of a "let it happen" nature called "passive concentration."

Progressive Relaxation emphasizes the relaxation of voluntary skeletal muscles—that is, all muscles over which you have conscious control. This technique seeks to achieve increased control over skeletal muscle until a subject is able to induce very low levels of tension in the major muscle groups, such as in the arms and legs. Dr. E. Jacobson, a physiologist-physician who devised the technique, argues that anxiety neurosis and other related diseases are caused or aggravated by skeletal muscle contraction, whereas muscular relaxation produces opposite physiologic states. Progressive relaxation is practiced lying down in a quiet room; a passive attitude is essential because mental images induce slight, measurable muscle tension, especially in the eyes and face. The subject is taught to recognize even these minute contractions of his or her muscles so that he or she can avoid them and achieve the deepest degree of relaxation possible.

Hypnosis, a more widely known but still poorly understood technique, may be defined as an altered state of consciousness which is artificially induced and characterized by increased receptiveness to suggestions. Thus, in the hypnotic state, a subject responding to the hypnotist's suggestion may feel hot, or raise his or her arm, or disregard pain, or temporarily lose all memory, or feel relaxed. The hypnotic induction procedure usually includes suggestions (auto-suggestions for self-hypnosis) of relaxation and drowsiness, closed eyes, and a comfortable position. Following the induction procedure, an appropriate suggestion is given for the desired mental or physical behavior. So far it has not been possible to find a specific set of physiologic changes that characterize the hypnotic state. Instead, the physiologic changes vary according to the suggested state. When deep relaxation is the suggested state to be achieved by hypnosis, the physiologic changes of the Relaxation Response may be evoked.

Sentic Cycles, devised by Dr. Manfred Clynes, a gifted pianist as well as a psychophysiological researcher, demonstrates the close relation between emotional states and predictable physiologic changes. A Sentic "Cycle" is composed of eight "sentic states," or self-induced emotional experiences. The sequence of states used by Clynes consists of: no emotion; anger; hate; grief; love; sex; joy; reverence. A subject practices a cycle by thinking the state, for example, anger. Each time a click is heard from a tape recorder, he or she responds with finger pressure on a key similar to a piano key. The finger pressure is recorded on a chart. Through continuous measurements of various bodily functions, Clynes has noted markedly different but predictable physiologic changes when the subject experiences and reacts to the various suggested emotional states. Changes consistent with the elicitation of the Relaxation Response have been noted during the imagined emotional experiences of reverence, love, and grief.

Not only do we find the use of the Relaxation Response in relaxation-therapy settings, but we also believe that it has been a part of the cultures of man throughout the ages. The next chapter provides an historical perspective of this concept by presenting descriptions of the subjective accounts and practices utilized over the ages to evoke the Relaxation Response.

5

The physiologic changes of the Relaxation Response are associated with what has been called an altered state of consciousness. The term "altered state of consciousness" has become increasingly popular in recent years through frequent appearance in scores of books and literally hundreds of articles, ranging from esoteric journals such as *Psychophysiology* to *The New York Times Magazine*. There have been many accounts of what a person experiences under altered states of his consciousness, including ecstasy, unity with a higher being, selflessness, calm serenity, or a synthesis of all of these feelings. What happens in an "altered state of consciousness"? When we speak of consciousness we should think of a continuum extending from relatively deep unconsciousness at one end to an extraordinary sensitivity at the other. The continuum passes from coma to sleep to drowsiness, to alertness, to hyperalertness. In this continuum, one of the levels of consciousness, we believe, is associated with the Relaxation Response. It is an *altered* state simply because we do not commonly experience it, and because it usually does not occur spontaneously; it must be consciously and purposefully evoked.

A way to achieve this altered state of consciousness associated with the Relaxation Response is through the practice of what has been called *meditation,* which was illustrated in the previous chapter. The term "meditation" is difficult for some people to grasp because it may connote exotic Eastern cults or Christian monks who spend most of their waking hours in monastery cells contemplating God. As Dr. Robert E. Ornstein points out in his book *The Psychology of Consciousness,* the Western "impersonal, objective scientific approach, with its exclusive emphasis on logic and analysis makes it difficult for most of us even to conceive of a psychology which could be based on the existence of another, intuitive gestalt mode of thought." The notion of attaining "altered consciousness" may seem to you like some mystic experience involving a deep philosophical or religious ritual, and therefore too much like a cult.

Age-Old Wisdom

The altered state of consciousness associated with the Relaxation Response has been routinely experienced in Eastern and Western cultures throughout all ages. Subjectively, the feelings associated with this altered state of consciousness have been described as ecstatic, clairvoyant, beautiful, and totally relaxing. Others have felt ease with the world, peace of mind, and a sense of well-being akin to that feeling experienced after a period of exercise but without the fatigue. Most describe their feelings as *pleasurable*. Despite the diversity of description, there appears to be a universal element of rising above the mundane senses, a feeling beyond that of common-day existence. Many authors have pointed out the similarities between Eastern and Western mysticism, and have emphasized a universality of certain impulses in the human mind. Indeed, the subjective accounts of practitioners of different meditative backgrounds are similar to many experiences depicted in religious, historical, and philosophical writings. We will attempt to show that the Relaxation Response has been experienced throughout history. We will do so by extracting methods described in various literatures, primarily religious. Some of these methods are thousands of years old. Our chief purpose is to illustrate the age-old universality of this altered state of consciousness by citing certain elements that appear to be necessary to evoke this experience, or "response." No technique can claim uniqueness.

This approach is not to be interpreted as viewing religion or philosophy in a mechanistic fashion. The ultimate purpose of any exercise to attain transcendent experience corresponds to the philosophy or religion in which it is used. For example, John of Ruysbroeck, a Flemish mystic in the thirteenth century, states that through

> *. . . inward exercises man feels a ghostly union with God. Whosoever then has, in his inward exercise, an imageless and free ascent unto his God, and means nought else but the glory of God, must taste of the goodness of God; and he must feel from within a true union with God. And in this union, the inward and spiritual life is made perfect; for in this union, the desirous power is perpetually enticed anew and stirred to new inward activity. And by each act, the spirit rises upwards to a new union.*

Or, according to the teachings of Buddha, meditational exercises will help one realize and experience perfected selflessness leading to a cessation of unhappiness and a state of peace. However, the experience of this altered state of consciousness is not dependent upon one philosophical or religious belief. William James, one of the fathers of modern psychology, expresses this view in *The Variety of Religious Experience:*

The fact is that the mystical feeling of enlargement, union and emancipation has no specific intellectual content whatever of its own. It is capable of forming matrimonial alliances with material furnished by the most diverse philosophies and theology, provided only they can find a place in their framework for its peculiar emotional mood.

Also, many of the contemplative techniques set forth in the writings of Christian mystics used their own experiences and techniques only as example. An anonymous monk writing in the fourteenth century states in *The Cloud of Unknowing*:

And if you think that the labor is great, then you may seek to develop special ways, tricks, private techniques, and spiritual devices by means of which you can put other thoughts away. And it is best to learn these methods from God by your own experience rather than from any man in this life. Although this is so, I will tell you what seems to me to be the best of these special ways. Test them and improve upon them if you can.

Hence, by selecting elements from various techniques which appear to be necessary for eliciting experiences of transcendence, we are not espousing a certain tradition or taking away the special meaning of any practice for the individual. Because of the variety of experiences and methods, a person may find that any one of many practices best suits his or her purpose. As William James aptly states: "To find religion is only one out of many ways of reaching unity; and the process of remedying inner incompleteness and reducing inner discord is a general psychological process."

Meditation: The Four Basic Elements

Most accounts of what we now call the Relaxation Response are subjective descriptions of deeply personal, unique experiences. However, there appear to be four basic elements underlying the elicitation of the Relaxation Response, regardless of the cultural source.

The first element is *a quiet environment*. One must "turn off" not only internal stimuli but also external distractions. A quiet room or a place of worship may be suitable. The nature mystics meditated outdoors.

The second element is *an object to dwell upon*. This object may be a word or sound repetition; gazing at a symbol; concentrating on a particular feeling. For example, directing one's attention to the repetition of a syllable will help clear the mind. When distracting thoughts do occur, one can return to this repetition of the syllable to help eliminate other thoughts.

The third element is *a passive attitude*. It is an emptying of all thoughts and distractions from one's mind. *A passive attitude appears to be the most essential factor in eliciting the Relaxation Response.* Thoughts, imagery, and feelings may drift into one's awareness. One should not concentrate on these perceptions but allow them to pass on. A person should not be concerned with how well he or she is doing.

The fourth element is *a comfortable position*. One should be in a comfortable posture that will allow an individual to remain in the same position for at least twenty minutes. Usually a sitting position is recommended. We believe the sitting, kneeling, squatting, swaying postures assumed in various forms of prayer have evolved to keep the practitioner from falling asleep. The desired altered state of consciousness is not sleep, but the same four elements will lead to sleep if the practitioner is lying down.

The first selections illustrating these four elements will be from Christian writers, most of whom have been labeled mystics. However, the term *mysticism* was not a common term until medieval times. Rather, the subject of these writings was *contemplation*, whose end point was direct union with God. Let us begin with St. Augustine (A.D. 354–430), who wrote during the first great period of theological controversy, a time marking the beginning of Western civilization.

Contemplation for St. Augustine was upon the un-

changeable—that is, on God, "the Light Unchangeable."
Dom Cuthbert Butler, in his book *Western Mysticism*,
states that St. Augustine does not designate his experience as union with God, as do the later Christian mystics,
although he expresses the idea of some kind of spiritual
contact. Preparation for contemplation according to St.
Augustine is *recollection*, a term later used by many Christian mystics, which corresponds with the idea of a passive
attitude. Recollection is an exercise of abstraction, of rec-
ollecting and gathering together thoughts ("memory")
and concentrating the mind. The object is to shut off the
mind from external thoughts and to produce a mental
solitude. St. Augustine speaks of recollection or the preparation for contemplation in the following passage from
Confessions:

> *So great is the force of memory, so great the force of
> life, even in the mortal life of man. What shall I do
> then, O thou my true life, my God? I will pass even
> beyond this power of mine which is called memory;
> yea I will pass beyond it, that I may approach unto
> Thee, O sweet Light.*

St. Augustine's work is a moving chronicle that describes his own intensely personal experiences. In addition to portraying their own subjective experiences, later
Christian mystics set forth various components of con-

templation which they thought would lead their readers to this particular state of consciousness.

The Cloud of Unknowing, a book written probably during the fourteenth century, provided practical advice for all individuals desiring "to be knit to God in spirit, in unity of love, and accordance of will." The author, a monk, most likely remained anonymous because he feared he would be accused of heresy. He believed religion allowed for independent inquiry and individual experience, which at that time were condemned by the church. In his book he wrote that man gained direct knowledge of God by losing all awareness of himself. Referring to his title, the author depicts a passive attitude as the way "to cover," or forget, all distractions: "Try to cover these thoughts with a thick cloud of forgetting as though they never existed neither for you nor for any other man. And if they continue to arise, continue to put them down."

He goes on to discuss the element of "dwelling upon" and advises that his readers can develop "special ways, tricks, private techniques, and spiritual devices" in order to achieve contemplation. One means is the use of a single syllable such as "God" or "love":

Choose whichever one you prefer, or if you like, choose another that suits your tastes, provided that it is of one syllable. And clasp this word tightly in your heart so that it never leaves it no matter what may happen. This word shall be your shield and your spear whether you ride in peace or in war. With this word you shall beat upon the cloud and the darkness, which are above you. With this word you shall strike down thoughts of every kind and drive them beneath the cloud of forgetting.

Germany in the fourteenth century produced a number of mystics. As in *The Cloud of Unknowing,* the essence of their mysticism was the belief that the individual could directly commune with God when he was in a state of perfect solitude. Martin Luther drew upon this doctrine of individual transcendence to God. Rudolph Otto, a prominent German theologian and philosopher, describes methods of prayer from Luther's book *How Man Should Pray, Meister Peter, the Barber,* written in 1534. To prepare for prayers of inward recollections, the true language of the heart, in which one concentrates solely upon God, one must achieve a passive attitude by dwelling upon an object. It is necessary to have "the heart free itself and become joyous" in order to prevent thoughts from intruding. For the object upon which one concentrates, Luther suggests the words of the Lord's Prayer, the Ten Commandments, the Psalms, or a number of the sayings of Christ or Paul.

Like the anonymous fourteenth-century monk and Martin Luther, Fray Francisco de Osuna, a monk writing in the sixteenth century, sets forth spiritual exercises for those wishing to obtain union with God. In his preface to *The Third Spiritual Alphabet,* Fray Francisco de Osuna defends recollection as a natural means by which man can rise to the knowledge of God, citing references from the teachings of the Bible. For Fray Francisco de Osuna the act of contemplation is the act of love for God. In his Sixth Treatise of *The Third Spiritual Alphabet,* he advocates a quiet environment by relating the custom of Christ, who would retreat to the desert:

> *Although these practices and others of the same kind are excellent, our Letter advises those who wish to make further progress and follow better things to accustom themselves to recollection, for they will thus imitate and follow our Lord, whose custom it was to go into the desert, where, alone and recollected, he could pray more secretly and spiritually to his and our heavenly Father.*

Later, he describes the element of a quiet environment as "the quiet that nature ordains before sleep is ordained by the devout soul for prayer."

This sixteenth-century monk elaborates on the passive attitude by describing the soul as mute and deaf to purposeful and spontaneous thoughts:

> *You must also know that the world is by nature deaf, which must be understood to mean in this case that*

the soul which is mute, not meditating on any subject, should also be deaf regarding thoughts which drag it down, and repress the senses with their many distractions. Therefore it is well that under this Letter should be included the two words dumb and deaf, for the one forbids the wandering thoughts we purposely encourage, and the other prevents those that would arise from our many occupations and levity.

Two methods of dwelling upon an object are suggested for recollection. One method is gazing, which can be accomplished even in a crowd:

I do not tell you simply to lower your eyes, but to keep them fixed steadily on the ground, like men who are forgetful and as it were out of themselves, who stand immovable, wrapt in thought. Some people find it more easy to be recollected if they keep their eyes shut, but in order to avoid remark, it is better when in company to keep our gaze fixed on the ground, on some place where there is little to look at so that there may be less to stir our fancy and imagination. Thus, even in a crowd you may be deeply recollected by keeping your gaze bent, fixed on one place. The smaller and darker the place, the more limited your view will be and the less will your heart be distracted.

The second exercise is to repeat "no" when distracting thoughts occur:

> *If you wish to acquire recollection by practicing this holy exercise, remember to make use of a very brief means of ridding yourself of various distracting thoughts. This is that you say "No" to them when they come to you during prayer.*

Fray Francisco de Osuna continues and expands this idea of using the word "no" as a means of maintaining a passive attitude. When thoughts do occur during recollection one should not ponder whether they are signals from God:

> *I warn you against discussing the matter further in your mind; it would greatly disturb your recollection; to examine into the matter would be a hindrance; therefore, shut the door with "no." You will know that the Lord will come and enter your soul if the doors, which are your senses, are closed . . . But you will answer that it would be wrong to say "no" to God and he alone is expected. But God comes in some other way of which you know nothing.*

St. Teresa was very much influenced by Fray Francisco's writings on recollection. In 1562 she wrote *The Way* to *Perfection* to teach her fellow Sisters the habit of recollection:

> *May the Lord teach this manner of prayer to those who do not know it for I confess, myself, that I never knew what it was to pray with satisfaction until he instructed me in this method.*

To St. Teresa, a passive attitude is the soul's transcendence of earthly things:

> *. . . so the soul raises herself to a loftier region; she withdraws her senses from exterior objects . . . those who adopt this method almost always pray with their eyes shut . . . because it is making an effort not to think about earthly things.*

Although some call pure contemplation the prayer of the quiet, St. Teresa contends that many persons are raised to high contemplation by vocal prayers. An acquaintance was much distressed because she could not pray mentally:

> *[She] could never make any but vocal prayer, and, faithful to this, she had everything. Yet if she did not recite the words, her thoughts wandered so much that she could not bear it. But would that all had such*

mental prayer . . . I saw, that faithful to the Paternoster, she had reached pure contemplation.

On Mt. Athos, a peninsula of Greece, a traveler may still find monasteries that have remained essentially unchanged since the thirteenth century. The primitive Christianity of Mt. Athos represents the Eastern Orthodox Church at the time of the split between the Western and Eastern churches. In the late nineteen-fifties three men documented the lives of the monks living on Mt. Athos. In the following passage Father Nicolas discusses the hermit's life and explains how after isolating oneself from the world one must also abstract himself from his body and mind:

After years in a monastery or in a skete, detaching oneself from the world, the difficulty lies just in finding oneself alone, face to face with oneself, alone in control of your body and your mind. Because the mind is a wanderer, you know. Thoughts never stop following each other through your head, buzzing, preventing concentration, while in order to pray you need a great emptiness in your mind. After you've hunted out and punished all your vices, passions, faults— however trivial—you have to hunt out all your thoughts. You have to create an immense silence round you before you can reach the deepest silence in the depths of yourself. Continual prayer, repeating the same words of praise to the Lord; that's what allows one to pray. It's not a question of seeing God, but of being in God, and it's not easy to contain in the narrow limits of your body the limitless spirit which is always trying to escape. That's a hermit's life, more or less.

The repetition of words of praise to God is a form of prayer called Prayer of the Heart or Prayer of Jesus. It is a method of Hesychasm, which was adopted by Russian mysticism and developed at Mt. Athos. The Prayer of the Heart was often used as a method of contemplation in Russian monasticism. It was also used by devout lay people especially among the poor peasantry. The philosophical basis for the Prayer of the Heart dates back to the Greeks and St. Gregory Palamas, who believed that after the body and intellect are purified man can regain intuitive wisdom, as before the fall of mankind depicted by Adam. The method of repetitive prayer purifies the intellect by means of a passive attitude, emptying it of all thought, image, and passion. A compendium of the writings of Greek fathers and the masters of Byzantine spirituality, the Philokalia, contains extensive writings concerning the Prayer of the Heart. All four elements of a quiet environment, a proper posture, a dwelling upon an object, and a passive attitude are found in the Philokalia:

Sit down alone and in silence. Lower your head, shut your eyes, breathe out gently, and imagine yourself looking into your own heart. As you breathe out, say "Lord Jesus Christ, have mercy on me." Say it, moving your lips gently, or simply say it in your mind. Try to put all other thoughts aside. Be calm, be patient and repeat the process very frequently.

The invocation should be timed to the rhythm of breathing:

You know, brother, how we breathe, we breathe the air in and out. On this is based the life of the body and on this depends its warmth. So, sitting down in your cell, collect your mind, lead it into the path of the breath along which the air enters in, constrain it to enter the heart altogether with inhaled air, and keep it there. Keep it there, but do not leave it silent and idle, instead give it the following prayer: "Lord, Jesus Christ, Son of God, have mercy upon me." Let this be its constant occupation, never to be abandoned. For this work, by keeping the mind free from dreaming, renders it unassailable to suggestions of the enemy and leads it to Divine desire and love. . . .

In the Judaic literature, one also finds portrayals of contemplative or meditative exercises. As in other religious literatures, the end purpose here is union with God.

The earliest form of mysticism in Judaism is Merkabol-ism, which dates back approximately to the first century A.D., the time of the Second Temple. Practices of this sect included various forms of asceticism, including fasting. Merkabolism's meditative exercises focused on body posture and the dwelling upon hymns and a magic emblem. The meditator would place his head between his knees and whisper hymns and repeat the name of a magic emblem. Repetition of the magic emblem was used as the object to dwell upon and would chase away distractions and cause the "demons and hostile angels to flight." A state of ecstasy was reached, which Gershom G. Scholem, a scholar of Jewish mysticism, has described as "an attitude of deep self-oblivion."

Writings on the techniques of mysticism in Judaism were prevalent in the thirteenth century. Many of the exercises involved dwelling upon the names of God or contemplating the letters constituting the name of God. Rabbi Abulafia developed such a mystical system of meditating upon letters of the Hebrew alphabet as constituents of God's name. The aim of his mystical theory was to "unseal the soul, to untie the knots which bind it." Kept within the limits defined by one's sensory perceptions and emotions, the soul's life is finite, for these limits are finite. Hence, man needs a higher form of perception which, rather than blocking the soul's deeper regions, will open them up. This perception must be capable of the highest importance without having any importance of its own. In order to accomplish this, one needs an absolute object upon which to meditate. Thus, Rabbi Abulafia used the letters of God's name because the name is absolute. It reflects the meaning and totality of existence, yet to the human mind has no concrete meaning of its own.

Gershom G. Scholem characterizes Abulafia's teaching as similar to Yoga, whose meditative techniques will be discussed in a moment. He writes that Abulafia's

> . . . *teachings represent but a Judaized version of that ancient spiritual technique which has found its classical expression in the practices of the Indian mystics who follow the system known as* Yoga. *To cite only one instance out of many, an important part in Abulafia's system is played by the technique of breathing; now this technique has found its highest development in the Indian* Yoga, *where it is commonly regarded as the most important instrument of mental discipline. Again, Abulafia lays down certain rules of body posture, certain corresponding combinations of consonants and vowels, and certain forms of recitation, and in particular some passages of his book* "The Light of the Intellect" *give the impression of a Judaized treatise on* Yoga. *The similarity even extends to some aspects of the doctrine of ecstatic vision, as preceded and brought about by these practices.*

In the East, meditative practices have perhaps had a more pervasive role not only in its religions but also in its cultural traditions. Carolyn Spurgeon, a professor of English literature, in an essay on mysticism in English literature points out an interesting difference between Eastern and Western mysticism. Western mysticism, she writes, stemmed from the Greek delight in natural beauty and reached its fullest development with the teachings of Christian faith. Enlightenment in Christianity centered upon the doctrine of Incarnation, in which the mystery of God would reveal itself in human form. Hence, Spurgeon concludes, Western mystical thought has embodied all that is human and natural, of human love and intellect and of the natural world. To Eastern thinking, however, this "humanness" obstructs spiritual ascent. The emphasis of Eastern mysticism has been on pure soul-consciousness, to annihilate the flesh and deny its reality in order to reach absolute freedom.

Yoga has been a tradition in India throughout its history. Not merely a philosophy, Yoga has influenced many different practices and beliefs throughout the Indian culture. Mircea Eliade has traced the doctrines and methods of Yoga which have permeated numerous Eastern religions and philosophies—Brahmanism, the Upanishads of Vedic literature, Hinduism, Buddhism, Tantrism, to name a few. Eliade's definition of Yoga is any ascetic technique and method of meditation. The "classic" system of Yoga can be found in the writings of Patañjali, who brought together and classified a series of traditional practices and contemplative formulas. The essence of Yoga meditation is concentration on a single point—for example, a physical object or a thought. By dwelling upon an object one may cancel out all distractions that are associated with one's everyday life and thus achieve a passive attitude. Eliade describes this concentration, *ekā-gratā*, as damming the mental stream of the mind. *Ekā-gratā*, or concentration, may be reached through numerous techniques such as decreased muscle tone and rhythmic breathing. By means of these techniques one may attain *ekāgratā* and ultimately the highest concentration, *samādhi*, in which one passes beyond the human condition to total freedom.

H. Saddhatissa, in his presentation of Buddhism for Western readers, outlines methods for the practice of meditation which parallel Eliade's description of Yoga techniques. Buddhism, whose philosophy is attributed to Siddhārtha Gautama (?563-?483 B.C.), began in the northern province of India. At one time Buddhism prevailed throughout Asia, and for twenty-five centuries it has been part of traditional beliefs in many lands. Saddhatissa estimates there are five hundred million Buddhists in India, Nepal, China, Japan, Korea, Tibet, Cambodia, Laos, Vietnam, Malaysia, Myanmar, Thailand, and Ceylon. The preliminary instructions that Saddhatissa presents for meditation include a quiet environment and a comfortable position. One should choose a suitable place, which will have few distractions and therefore help one concentrate. He suggests a sitting posture, not necessarily a lotus, cross-legged, position, but a position that one finds comfortable.

Saddhatissa proceeds from these preparations to categorize two types of Buddhist meditation—*samatha*, the development of calm and concentration, and *vispassanā*, the development of insight. In *samatha* the meditator concentrates on a fixed object, either external or internal. *Ānāpānasati*, one of the foremost practices of *samatha*, was used by the Buddha on the night of his enlightenment. It is the practice of in-breathing and out-breathing. Focusing his attention at the tip of his nostrils, the meditator quietly "watches" the breath flowing in and out past the tip of the nostril. It is recommended that he count breaths, not going past ten, and repeating the count to aid his concentration.

Ashvagosha, an eminent Buddhist of the first century A.D., formulated and expounded the teachings of the Mahayana school, a more elaborate and developed form of the original doctrines of Buddhism. Ashvagosha's book *The Awakening of Faith* instructs the reader how to practice the Mahayana faith. The practice consists of five stages, the fifth being the "stage of preventing vain thoughts, and the practice of divine wisdom or judgments." These two concepts are to be gradually activated at the same time. The practice of checking vain thoughts is accomplished through a quiet environment, a proper posture, and a passive attitude:

As to the practice of checking vain thoughts, it should be done in a quiet place, properly seated and in a proper spirit . . . for all kinds of ideas as soon as thought of must be put away, even the idea of banishing them must also be put away. As all existence originally came to be without any idea of its own, it ceases to be also without any idea of its own; any thoughts arising therefore must be from being absolutely passive. Nor must one follow the mind in its excursions to everything outside itself and then chase that thought away. If the mind wanders far away, it must be brought back into its proper state. One should know that the proper state is that of the soul alone without anything outside of it.

Eventually the practitioner will perfect this practice and the mind will be at rest, from which one will proceed to reach the "peace of the Eternal."

In the practices of Sufism, a system of Muhammadan mysticism, one discovers all of the four elements that together may bring about transcendent experiences. Muhammadanism was founded by Muhammad, the Arab prophet, who lived in the sixth century. However, the origins of the practices of Sufism may be traced back to the second century, and it is of interest to note its similarities to Christianity and Buddhism. Al-Ghazali, who has been described as the greatest Muslim since Muhammad, found the true way of life through Sufism although he remained an orthodox Muhammadan. Dhikr, a special method of worship in Sufism, is explained by Al-Ghazali in a passage that has been summarized by D. B. Macdonald and cited in *A Moslem Seeker After God* as follows:

Let the worshipper reduce his heart to a state in which the existence of anything and its nonexistence are the same to him. Then let him sit alone in some corner, limiting his religious duties to what is absolutely necessary, and not occupying himself either with reciting the Koran or considering its meaning or with books of religious traditions or with anything of the sort. And let him see to it that nothing save God most High enters his mind. Then, as he sits in solitude, let him not cease saying continuously with his tongue, "Allah, Allah," keeping his thought on it. At last he will reach a state when the motion of his tongue will cease, and it will seem as though the word flowed from it. Let him persevere in this until all trace of motion is removed from his tongue, and he finds his heart persevering in the thought. Let him still persevere until the form of the word, its letters and shape, is removed from his heart, and there remains the idea alone, as though clinging to his heart, inseparable from it. So far, all is dependent on his will and choice; but to bring the mercy of God does not stand in his will or choice. He has now laid himself bare to the breathings of that mercy, and nothing remains but to wait for what God will open to him, as God has done after this manner to prophets and saints. If he follows the above course, he may be sure that the light of the Real will shine out in his heart.

Taoism, one of the influential philosophical systems in the history and thought of China, dates back to the sixth century B.C., with the writing of *Lao Tzu,* which embodies all of Taoist philosophy. Chuang Tzu, who lived two hundred years later, elaborated upon the teachings of *Lao Tzu,* developing more clearly the concepts of Taoism and placing a stronger emphasis on the individual. To practice Taoism, according to Chuang Tzu, is "To regard the fundamental as the essence, to regard things as coarse, to regard accumulation as deficiency, and to dwell quietly alone with the spiritual and the intellect—herein lie the techniques of Tao of the ancients. . . . They built their doctrines on the principle of the eternal non-being and held the idea of the Great One as fundamental." Through tranquillity of mind one achieves accord with nature and hence with Tao, the "One." Chuang Tzu says that dwelling quietly alone with the spirit and the intellect means "forgetting everything," much as the author of *The Cloud of Unknowing* instructs the reader to cover thoughts with a "thick cloud of forgetting." Chuang Tzu presents the following passage:

Yen Hui said, "I have made some progress."

"What do you mean?" asked Confucius.

*"I have forgotten humanity and righteousness,"
replied Yen Hui.*

*"Very good, but that is not enough," said
Confucius.*

*On another day Yen Hui saw Confucius again
and said, "I have made some progress."*

"What do you mean?" asked Confucius.

*"I have forgotten ceremonies and music," replied
Yen Hui.*

*"Very good, but that is not enough," said
Confucius.*

*Another day Yen Hui saw Confucius again and
said, "I have made some progress."*

"What do you mean?" asked Confucius.

*Yen Hui said, "I forget everything while sitting
down."*

*Confucius' face turned pale. He said, "What do
you mean by sitting down and forgetting everything?"*

*"I cast aside my limbs," replied Yen Hui, "dis-
card my intelligence, detach from both body and
mind, and become one with the Great Universal
[Tao]. This is called sitting down and forgetting
everything."*

*Confucius said, "When you become one with the
Great Universal, you will have no partiality, and
when you are part of the process of transformation,*

you will have no constancy. You are really a worthy man. I beg to follow your steps."

Yoga breathing techniques, as described earlier, were assimilated by religious Taoists. However, the concern of these exercises was the indefinite prolongation of life and the material body rather than the Indian philosophy of attaining spiritual transcendence. Eliade describes one Taoist technique of inner breathing as choosing a quiet room, loosening the hair, unfastening the clothes, and lying down in the right position. After harmonizing his breaths, the practitioner holds his breath until doing so becomes intolerable. During this time he must "darken the heart [the organ of thought] so it does not think." The procedure should then be repeated.

Similar meditative practices may be found in practically every culture. Shamanism, for example, is a form of mysticism in which a chant or song intoned by a Shaman, or holy man, brings on trances. Shamanism is practiced in conjunction with tribal religions in North and South America, Indonesia, Africa, Siberia, and Japan.

Also, meditative practices may be found outside of a religious or philosophical context, and a rich source of descriptions of transcendent experiences is secular literature. For many poets and writers these feelings were revelations of ecstasy. Carolyn Spurgeon in her book *Mysticism in English Literature* traces the influence of mysticism on eighteenth- and nineteenth-century poets.

Of particular interest are Brontë, Wordsworth, and Tennyson. Spurgeon describes Emily Brontë's poems as strong and free, isolated from any dogma and containing the simplest language, portraying the record of the experience and the vision of the soul. In "The Prisoner" the element of a passive attitude is rapturously recounted as the loss of outward senses.

> *He comes with western winds, with evening's wandering airs.*
> *With that clear dusk of heaven that brings the thickest stars.*
> *Winds take a pensive tone, and stars a tender fire,*
> *And visions rise, and change, that kill me with desire.*
>
> *But, first, a hush of peace—a soundless calm descends;*
> *The struggle of distress, and fierce impatience ends;*
> *Mute music soothes my breast—unuttered harmony,*
> *That I could never dream, till Earth was lost to me.*
>
> *Then dawns the Invisible; the Unseen its truth reveals;*
> *My outward sense is gone, my inward essence feels;*
> *Its wings are almost free—its home, its harbour found,*
> *Measuring the gulf, it stoops and dares the final bound.*
>
> *Oh! dreadful is the check—intense the agony—*
> *When the ear begins to hear, and the eye begins to see;*

When the pulse begins to throb, the brain to think again;
The soul to feel the flesh, and the flesh to feel the chain.

Wordsworth believed that every man could attain the vision of joy and harmony of life in nature, which for him transformed the whole of existence. Spurgeon calls his poetry a series of notes and investigations devoted to the practical and detailed explanation of how this state of vision might be reached. Wordsworth's description of the method of realizing this condition emphasizes the practice of a passive attitude. If freed from distracting objects, petty cares, "little enmities and low desires," he could reach an equilibrium of "wise passiveness" or a "happy stillness of the mind." A cessation of the intellect and desires and a relaxation of the will could be used deliberately to induce this condition. With habitual training one could experience the "central peace subsisting for ever at the heart of endless agitation." He describes this experience in the following lines from "Tintern Abbey."

. . . *that serene and blessed mood,*
In which . . . the breath of this corporeal frame,
And even the motion of our human blood,
Almost suspended, we are laid asleep
In body, and become a living soul:
While with an eye made quiet by the power
Of harmony, and the deep power of joy,
We see into the life of things.

Tennyson had peculiar experiences of a vision of ecstasy which was the foundation of his deepest beliefs of the "unity of all things, the reality of the unseen, and the persistence of life." This condition came about often with the silent repetition of his own name! He wrote several accounts of this experience:

> . . . *till all at once, as it were, out of the intensity of the consciousness of individuality, the individuality itself seemed to resolve and fade away into boundless being, and this not a confused state, but the clearest of the clearest, the surest of the surest, utterly beyond words, where death was an almost laughable impossibility, the loss of personality (if so it were) seeming no extinction, but the only true life.*

In sum, there appear to be certain common elements in almost all cultures which enable individuals to periodically change their everyday mode of thinking. We believe this mental process is accompanied by the previously described physiologic changes of the Relaxation Response. Our usual thinking is concerned with events outside ourselves. Through our emotional attachments, our social feelings, our ideological beliefs, our sensory contacts, we are constantly diverting our thinking toward external factors. Any attempt to redirect this outwardly directed consciousness requires a different mental process. We believe that people have been describing the type of thinking which elicits the Relaxation Response throughout many cultures and religions. Until recently most observers were concerned only with the philosophical and subjective aspects of the Relaxation Response. The accompanying physiologic changes were probably not of interest. If they were, they could not have been measured until modern technology was available.

6

.

Decreasing Blood Pressure

We have pointed out that the regular inappropriate activation of the fight-or-flight response may lead to such
diseases as hypertension with its often deadly consequences of heart attacks and strokes. We have also shown
that a response opposite to the fight-or-flight response
resides within all of us. Because the Relaxation Response
counteracts the arousal of the fight-or-flight response, it
is not unreasonable to expect that the regular evocation
of the Relaxation Response might lead to lower blood

pressure in patients *who already have high blood pressure.* We are aware, of course, that nondrug approaches to the treatment of high blood pressure, such as rest, are not original. But the Relaxation Response as such has not been previously used in therapy. To consider the Relaxation Response as an adjunctive therapeutic tool to those which already exist is a new concept.

An initial investigation was designed to test the hypothesis: does the regular evocation of the Relaxation Response have a place in the therapy of patients who already have high blood pressure? Transcendental Meditation was used as the mode of eliciting the Relaxation Response, since at the beginning of this investigation other techniques had not yet been fully tested. We were, however, comfortable with Transcendental Meditation and had the complete support and cooperation of the T.M. organization. I conducted the investigation in collaboration with B. R. Marzetta, B. A. Rosner, and H. P. Klemchuk. Four centers of the International Meditation Society which taught Transcendental Meditation served as a resource for providing subjects and for the measurements made. Would-be initiates of Transcendental Meditation were asked if they had high blood pressure, and if they did whether they would be willing to participate in a study of the effects of meditation on high blood pressure in exchange for not having to pay the T.M. initiation fee. Eighty-six subjects volunteered and were accepted. They agreed to put off learning meditation for six weeks while their blood pressure was periodically measured and recorded to establish their pre-meditation blood pressures. They were told to stay under their doctors' care and change their medications only if they were told to do so by their doctors.

Because blood pressure varies considerably even within a single individual, scores of measurements were taken for each individual over the six-week period. To eliminate possible observer bias, a special machine was used which muddles the numbers and deciphers them only after the measurement has been made. Thus, the person doing the measuring of blood pressure did not know the subject's true blood pressure even when actually making the measurement. At the end of the six-week period, the volunteers were taught how to activate the Relaxation Response through the practice of Transcendental Meditation.

Once the volunteers were regularly evoking the Relaxation Response, they were again repeatedly measured at random periods of the day, *but never while meditating.* They returned approximately every two weeks for their blood pressure measurements and were also asked several questions. What antihypertensive medications were they taking? What other medications were they taking? How had their diets changed? Had their smoking habits changed? How regularly did they practice meditation?

Out of the group of over eighty people, only thirty-six had not changed their antihypertensive medications or had never taken such medication in the first place. Others, for various reasons, had altered their medications and were dropped from the study lest the results reflect the effects of altered medication and not the effects of meditation. For the remaining thirty-six subjects comparisons were made between blood pressures prior to learning meditation and blood pressures after regularly eliciting the Relaxation Response through Transcendental Meditation.

During the pre-meditation control period, the systolic blood pressure (the highest component of blood pressure) of these thirty-six subjects averaged 146 millimeters of mercury. After several weeks of regularly practicing the Relaxation Response, the average systolic blood pressure decreased to 137. The 137 millimeters of mercury level represents a drop of about ten millimeters of mercury, lowering the blood pressure from the borderline high blood pressure range to the "normal" range. These changes are of statistical significance; that is, it is extremely improbable that they are due to chance. The average diastolic pressure (the lowest component of blood pressure) of this same group of thirty-six dropped from 93.5 to 88.9, again a change from the borderline high blood pressure range to the "normal" range. These changes were also statistically significant. We observed, moreover, that the decreases in blood pressure occurred during periods of the day unrelated to the meditation. As long as the subjects continued to meditate regularly for two brief periods a day, their blood pressures stayed measurably lower. But the meditation had not *cured* them. The subjects' lower blood pressure readings lasted only as long as they practiced the Relaxation Response regularly. When three of the ten subjects with the highest systolic and four of the ten subjects with the highest diastolic blood pressures chose to *stop* the regular practice of Transcendental Meditation, their blood pressures returned to their initial hypertensive levels within four weeks.

Which physiologic factors that control blood pressure are altered during meditation? Our hypothesis is that the Relaxation Response *decreases* and *counteracts* the increased sympathetic nervous system activity that accompanies the arousal of the fight-or-flight response. This sympathetic nervous system activity is reflected in the measures, reported in Chapter 4, of oxygen consumption, heart rate, respiratory rate, and blood pressure, which increase with the fight-or-flight response and decrease with the elicitation of the Relaxation Response.

This is one of the first studies in which the regular activation of the Relaxation Response has been tested in a group of hypertensive subjects, and it suggests a new approach to the therapy of hypertension, or high blood pressure. What we have presented are early results that are now being retested in other laboratories. Some of these other laboratories have already verified these findings.

The risks of developing the atherosclerotic diseases, as pointed out in Chapter 2, are directly related to the level of blood pressure, and anything that lowers blood pressure without undue side effects is beneficial. Prescribed drugs that decrease blood pressure are therefore very effective therapy. Standard medical therapy means taking antihypertensive drugs, which often act by interrupting the activity of the sympathetic nervous system, thus lowering blood pressure. The pharmacologic method of lowering blood pressure is very effective and extremely important since, to again emphasize, lowered blood pressure leads to a lower risk of developing atherosclerosis and its related diseases such as heart attacks and strokes. The regular practice of the Relaxation Response is yet another way to lower blood pressure. Indications are that this response affects the same mechanisms and lowers blood pressure by the same means as some antihypertensive drugs. Both counteract the activity of the sympathetic nervous system. It is unlikely that the regular elicitation of the Relaxation Response by itself will prove to be adequate therapy for severe or moderate high blood pressure. Probably it would act to enhance the lowering of blood pressure along with antihypertensive drugs, and thus lead to the use of fewer drugs or a lesser dosage. In the case of mild hypertension, the regular evocation of the Relaxation Response may be of great value, since it has none of the pharmacologic side effects often present with drugs and might possibly supplant their use. *But no matter how encouraging these initial results, no person should treat himself for high blood pressure by regularly eliciting the Relaxation Response. You should always do so under the care of your physician, who will routinely monitor your blood pressure to make sure it is adequately controlled.*

In brief, then, this initial controlled experiment shows that blood pressure can be lowered in hypertensive subjects through the use of the Relaxation Response. This experiment gives added weight to the concept that hypertension may be due in part to situations that require behavioral adjustment, since hypertension was alleviated by a behavioral technique, the regular use of the Relaxation Response. If high blood pressure can be alleviated by behavioral means alone, its cause may also lie in a behavioral mechanism.

By far the most appealing use of the Relaxation Response in relation to hypertension lies in its preventive aspects. To establish the preventive role of the Relaxation Response in hypertension, it is necessary to conduct large, expensive, and difficult investigations that often take many years to complete. We hope that such preventive studies may be started in the not-too-distant future.

The Relaxation Response serves as a *natural* way to counteract increased sympathetic nervous system activity associated with the fight-or-flight response. This means that the Relaxation Response should be useful in alleviating other disease states where increased sympathetic nervous system activity is a principal factor in the development of the disease or is an undesirable accompanying factor of that disease. For example, research is currently being carried out to test the usefulness of the Relaxation Response in alleviating various anxiety states. The usefulness of the Relaxation Response in treating the cardiac problem of dangerous, irregular heartbeats is also being tested.

Decreasing Drug Use

Another area of the therapeutic use of the Relaxation Response has been drug abuse. It had been claimed that people who elicit the Relaxation Response through Transcendental Meditation use fewer drugs. To test the validity of these claims Dr. R. K. Wallace and I conducted a study in collaboration with C. Dahl and D. F. Cook. Questionnaires were distributed to almost two thousand people who were training to be teachers of Transcendental Meditation. Approximately one thousand males and eight hundred females responded, ranging in age from fourteen to seventy-eight, with more than half the subjects in the nineteen-to-twenty-three-year-old range. Most of the participants had attended college, and many had received college degrees. On the average, they had been practicing meditation for about twenty months. (At least three months of the regular practice of meditation was required for participation in the study.) The subjects were asked to recall their drug-use habits before starting meditation and were then classified as nonusers, light, medium, and heavy users for various drug categories, including marijuana, hashish, amphetamines, LSD, other hallucinogens, narcotics, barbiturates, and hard liquor. Cigarette use was also noted.

In the six-month period prior to starting the practice of meditation, slightly over 1,450 participants in the study (78 percent) had used marijuana and hashish or both, and of that group 28 percent were classified as heavy users (once a day or more). After practicing Transcendental Meditation for about six months, only 37 percent reported they used marijuana. These figures indicate that over 40 percent discontinued their use of drugs after the intervention of Transcendental Meditation. After twenty-one months of regular practice, only 12 percent continued to use marijuana, a decrease of 66 percent. Of those who still used drugs, most were light users; only one individual was classified as a heavy user.

The decrease in use of LSD was even more marked. Before starting the practice of Transcendental Meditation, approximately nine hundred people, or nearly one-half of the participants, had used LSD. Of this group, 433 were medium or heavy users (that is, used the drug one to three times per month or more). During the first three months of meditation, 233 people continued to use

LSD, while after twenty-two months 97 percent of LSD users had given up the drug.

Decreases also occurred in the use of other hallucinogens (mescaline, peyote, STP, DMT), amphetamines, and narcotics. Prior to meditating, 39 percent were users of these other hallucinogens. After meditating for twenty-two to thirty-three months, only 4 percent were users. Thirty-two percent used amphetamines prior to starting meditation, and after the same time span of twenty-two to thirty-three months only 1 percent were users. Seventeen percent used narcotics, including heroin, opium, morphine, and cocaine, before, and 1 percent after the twenty-two– to thirty-three–month period.

It would appear that the regular practice of meditation in this highly select group of people did, in fact, lead to decreased drug use. Student drug users are, as a group, knowledgeable about the undesirable effects of drug abuse. In general, it is not difficult for most to stop; the problem is getting them to want to stop. Perhaps the regular use of the Relaxation Response can provide a nonchemical alternative to fulfill at least some of the basic motivations behind student drug abuse. From the questionnaire it became apparent that not only did the subjects stop using drugs, but they also dropped off in the active selling of drugs and changed their attitude to the extent of actually discouraging others from using drugs. They claimed drugs interfered with the profound feelings that accompanied meditation, which they enjoyed more than the highs or lows of drugs.

In the same questionnaire, the participants were asked about their hard-liquor intake (not wine or beer) and cigarette-smoking habits. Before the regular practice of meditation was begun, 60 percent of the participants used hard liquor and, of these, about 4 percent were heavy users (that is, drank hard liquor once a day or more). After twenty-one months of meditation, approximately 25 percent used hard liquor and only 0.1 percent were heavy users.

Approximately 48 percent smoked cigarettes before starting meditation and 27 percent were heavy users (more than one pack a day). Marked decreases were seen after twenty-one months of practicing Transcendental Meditation: 16 percent smoked cigarettes and only 5.8 percent were heavy users. The results were preliminary and uncontrolled, but still showed decreased alcohol intake and cigarette smoking with the use of the Relaxation Response.

The drug-use study had weaknesses. First, it dealt only with people who were actively pursuing meditation while the study was under way and who planned to continue to meditate. What we do not know is how many people started meditation and gave it up, only to go back to drugs. There was another bias. The subjects, as teachers of Transcendental Meditation, had a vested interest in the study. It was also a retrospective study. People were asked to remember what their drug-abuse habits had been previously, and the recollection of these habits left room for exaggeration and distortion of the actual amount of drugs used.

To deal with these limitations and other biases, we established a large prospective study in collaboration with Dr. Maynard W. Shelley, of the University of Kansas. It was prospective in that it noted drug-abuse habits as they developed from the beginning to the end of the study. This prospective-study design did away with the problems of recollection inherent in retrospective studies. This study was conducted at selected high schools in Massachusetts and Michigan, where junior-year students were asked, after being assured of anonymity, to fill out a questionnaire assessing their drug-abuse habits and their various psychological traits. Then individual high schools were matched with respect to size and geographic proximity. Programs of Transcendental Meditation were introduced in half of the matched high schools. The other matched schools were not presented with the introductory courses. In these high schools, there were several thousand students who answered questionnaires covering their drug-use habits and their willingness to learn Transcendental Meditation. Only thirty-six chose to learn T.M. Of those who did learn, only six practiced regularly. Those who did practice regularly used fewer drugs and confirmed the previous findings. However, Transcendental Meditation was apparently not an acceptable technique among the high-school students tested. Perhaps other techniques eliciting the Relaxation Response would have been more easily adapted to these students' life-styles and thus more readily accepted and practiced.

So far, we have been speaking positively of the Relaxation Response, of the way it may be applied to combat hypertension and also of its potential use in dealing with drugs, alcoholism, and cigarette smoking. Yet the regular practice of the Relaxation Response does not invariably produce results and should not be considered a panacea. For example, in another prospective study, which I conducted in collaboration with Dr. John R. Graham of the Headache Foundation, Inc., of Boston, and Helen P. Klemchuk, people kept daily records of the amount of medication they took as well as the frequency and severity of their headaches prior to the regular practice of Transcendental Meditation. They continued to keep these daily records while they regularly practiced the technique. The investigation showed that among seventeen patients suffering from *severe migraine* headache, only three were helped by the regular elicitation of the Relaxation Response associated with Transcendental Meditation. One of the seventeen was actually made worse, and the remaining thirteen showed no significant change in the number of headaches they had or in the amount of medication they took prior to and during the regular elicitation of the response.

Not long ago, the treatment of polio involved hundreds of millions of dollars. Then, in the space of several years, Nobel laureate Dr. John F. Enders conducted experiments in which the poliomyelitis virus was cultured in human kidney cells. The subsequent production of the Salk and Sabine vaccines turned the enormous financial costs of the disease, aside from the costs in personal suffering, into the relatively inexpensive price of immunization and in the process effectively wiped out polio from modern society. Similarly, the prevention of stress-related diseases carries with it enormous significance, certainly for the individual and his family in terms of their own physical and mental well-being, and for society as a whole through huge dollar savings in health expenditures. It is possible that the regular elicitation of the Relaxation Response will prevent the huge personal suffering and social costs now being inflicted on us by high blood pressure and its related ailments.

7
.

The case for the use of the Relaxation Response by healthy but harassed individuals is straightforward. It can act as a built-in method of counteracting the stresses of everyday living which bring forth the fight-or-flight response. We have also shown how the Relaxation Response may be used as a new approach to aid in the treatment and perhaps prevention of diseases such as hypertension. In this chapter, we will review the components necessary to evoke the Relaxation Response and present a specific technique that we have developed at Harvard's Thorndike Memorial Laboratory and Boston's Beth Israel Hospital. We again emphasize that, for those who may suffer from any disease state, the potential therapeutic use of the Relaxation Response should be practiced only under the care and supervision of a physician.

How to Bring Forth the Relaxation Response

In Chapter 5 we reviewed the Eastern and Western religious, cultic, and lay practices that led to the Relaxation Response. From those age-old techniques we have extracted four basic components necessary to bring forth that response:

(1) A Quiet Environment

Ideally, you should chose a quiet, calm environment with as few distractions as possible. A quiet room is suitable, as is a place of worship. The quiet environment contributes to the effectiveness of the repeated word or phrase by making it easier to eliminate distracting thoughts.

(2) A Mental Device

To shift the mind from logical, externally oriented thought, there should be a constant stimulus: a sound, word, or phrase repeated silently or aloud; or fixed gazing at an object. Since one of the major difficulties in the elicitation of the Relaxation Response is "mind wandering," the repetition of the word or phrase is a way to help break the train of distracting thoughts. Your eyes are usually closed if you are using a repeated sound or word; of course, your eyes are open if you are gazing. Attention to the normal rhythm of breathing is also useful and enhances the repetition of the sound or the word.

(3) A Passive Attitude

When distracting thoughts occur, they are to be disregarded and attention redirected to the repetition or gazing; *you should not worry about how well you are performing the technique,* because this may well prevent the Relaxation Response from occurring. Adopt a "let it happen" attitude. *The passive attitude is perhaps the most important element in eliciting the Relaxation Response. Distracting thoughts will occur. Do not worry about them. When these thoughts do present themselves and you become aware of them, simply return to the repetition of the mental device. These other thoughts do not mean you are performing the technique incorrectly. They are to be expected.*

(4) A Comfortable Position

A comfortable posture is important so that there is no undue muscular tension. Some methods call for a sitting position. A few practitioners use the cross-legged "lotus" position of the Yogi. If you are lying down, there is a tendency to fall asleep. As we have noted previously, the various postures of kneeling, swaying, or sitting in a cross-legged position are believed to have evolved to prevent falling asleep. You should be comfortable and relaxed.

It is important to remember that there is not a single method that is unique in eliciting the Relaxation Response. For example, Transcendental Meditation is one of the many techniques that incorporate these components. However, we believe it is not necessary to use the specific method and specific *secret,* personal sound taught by Transcendental Meditation. *Tests at the Thorndike Memorial Laboratory of Harvard have shown that a similar technique used with any sound or phrase or prayer or mantra brings forth the same physiologic changes noted during Transcendental Meditation:* decreased oxygen consumption; decreased carbon-dioxide elimination; decreased rate of breathing. In other words using the basic necessary components, any one of the age-old or the newly derived techniques produces the same physiologic results regardless of the mental device used. The following set of instructions, used to elicit the Relaxation Response, was developed by our group at Harvard's Thorndike Memorial Laboratory and was found to produce the same physiologic changes we had observed during the practice of Transcendental Meditation. This technique is now being used to lower blood pressure in certain patients. A non-cultic technique, it is drawn with little embellishment from the four basic components found in the myriad of historical methods. We claim no innovation but simply a scientific validation of age-old wisdom. The technique is our current method of eliciting the Relaxation Response in our continuing studies at the Beth Israel Hospital of Boston.

1. Sit quietly in a comfortable position.

2. Close your eyes.

3. Deeply relax all your muscles, beginning at your feet and progressing up to your face. Keep them relaxed.

4. Breathe through your nose. Become aware of your breathing. As you breathe out, say the word, "ONE," silently to yourself. For example, breathe IN . . . OUT, "ONE"; IN . . . OUT, "ONE"; etc. Breathe easily and naturally.

5. Continue for 10 to 20 minutes. You may open your eyes to check the time, but do not use an alarm. When you finish, sit quietly for several minutes, at first with your eyes closed and later with your eyes opened. Do not stand up for a few minutes.

6. Do not worry about whether you are successful in achieving a deep level of relaxation. Maintain a passive attitude and permit relaxation to occur at its own pace. When distracting thoughts occur, try to ignore them by not dwelling upon them and return to repeating "ONE." With practice, the response should come with little effort. Practice the technique once or twice daily, but not within two hours after any meal, since the digestive processes seem to interfere with the elicitation of the Relaxation Response.

The subjective feelings that accompany the elicitation of the Relaxation Response vary among individuals. The majority of people feel a sense of calm and feel very relaxed. A small percentage of people immediately experience ecstatic feelings. Other descriptions that have been related to us involve feelings of pleasure, refreshment, and well-being. Still others have noted relatively little change on a subjective level. Regardless of the subjective feelings described by our subjects, we have found that the physiologic changes, such as decreased oxygen consumption, are taking place.

There is no educational requirement or aptitude necessary to experience the Relaxation Response. Just as each of us experiences anger, contentment, and excitement, each has the capacity to experience the Relaxation Response. It is an innate response within us. Again, there are many ways in which people bring forth the Relaxation

Response, and your own individual considerations may be applied to the four components involved. You may wish to use the technique we have presented but with a different mental device. You may use a syllable or phrase that may be easily repeated and sounds natural to you.

Another technique you may wish to use is a prayer from your religious tradition. Choose a prayer that incorporates the four elements necessary to bring forth the Relaxation Response. As we have shown in Chapter 5, we believe every religion has such prayers. We would reemphasize that we do not view religion in a mechanistic fashion simply because a religious prayer brings forth this desired physiologic response. Rather, we believe, as did William James, that these age-old prayers are one way to remedy an inner incompleteness and to reduce inner discord. Obviously, there are many other aspects to religious beliefs and practices which have little to do with the Relaxation Response. However, there is little reason not to make use of an appropriate prayer within the framework of your own beliefs if you are most comfortable with it.

Your individual considerations of a particular technique may place different emphasis upon the components necessary to elicit the Relaxation Response and also may incorporate various practices into the use of the technique. For example, for some a quiet environment with little distraction is crucial. However, others prefer to practice the Relaxation Response in subways or trains. Some people choose always to practice the Relaxation Response in the same place and at a regular time.

Since the daily use of the Relaxation Response necessitates a slight change in life-style, some find it difficult at first to keep track of the regularity with which they evoke the Response. In our investigations of the Relaxation Response, patients use the calendar reprinted for your convenience on pages 144 and 145. Each time they practice the Relaxation Response, they make a check in the appropriate box.

It may be said, as an aside, that many people have told us that they use our technique for evoking the Relaxation Response while lying in bed to help them fall asleep. Some have even given up sleeping pills as a result. It should be noted, however, that when you fall asleep using the technique, you are not experiencing the Relaxation Response, you are asleep. As we have shown, the Relaxation Response is different from sleep.

Personal Experiences With the Relaxation Response

Several illustrations of how people include the practice of the Relaxation Response in their daily lives should answer the question that you may now be posing: "How do I find the time?" One businessman evokes the Relaxation

Response late in the morning for ten or fifteen minutes in his office. He tells his secretary that he's "in conference" and not to let in any calls. Traveling quite a bit, he often uses the Relaxation Response while on the airplane. A housewife practices the Relaxation Response after her husband and children have left for the day. In the late afternoon, before her husband comes home, she again evokes the response, telling her children not to disturb her for twenty minutes. Another woman, a researcher, usually awakes ten or twenty minutes earlier in the morning in order to elicit the Relaxation Response before breakfast. If she wakes up too late, she tries to take a "relaxation break" rather than a coffee break at work. She finds a quiet spot and a comfortable chair while her co-workers are out getting coffee. On the subway, a factory worker practices the Relaxation Response while commuting to and from work. He claims he has not yet missed his stop. A student uses the Relaxation Response between classes. Arriving fifteen minutes early, he uses the empty classroom and says he is not bothered by other students entering the room. If the classroom is in use, he simply practices the response sitting in the corridor.

The regular use of the Relaxation Response has helped these people to be more effective in their day-to-day living. The businessman feels he is "clearing the cobwebs" that have accumulated during the morning. He also states he often gets new perspectives on perplexing business problems. The housewife, before regularly eliciting the Relaxation Response, found it very difficult to face the prospects of preparing dinner and getting the family organized for another day. She now feels more energetic and enjoys her family more. The researcher no longer requires two cups of coffee in the morning to get started at work, and the factory worker notes he "unwinds" going home. The student says he is more attentive and hardly ever falls asleep during lectures. He even attributes better grades to his regular elicitation of the Relaxation Response.

The examples of when people practice the Relaxation Response are numerous. You must consider not only what times are practical but also when you feel the use of the Relaxation Response is most effective. We believe the regular use of the Relaxation Response will help you better deal with the distressing aspects of modern life by lessening the effects of too much sympathetic nervous system activation. By this increased control of your bodily reactions, you should become more able to cope with your uncertainties and frustrations.

The following two descriptions of people who have regularly used the Relaxation Response for specific problems show how they feel the Relaxation Response has been of help to them. A young man, who suffered from severe anxiety attacks, reports that he often felt fearful, nervous and shaky, tense and worried. After practicing the Relaxation Response for two months, he rarely suffered from attacks of anxiety. He felt considerably more calm and relaxed. Usually, he practiced the technique regularly twice a day, but he would also practice it when he began to feel anxious. By applying the technique in such a manner he found he could alleviate these oncoming feelings. In short, he felt that the practice of the Relaxation Response had significantly improved his life.

Our second illustration is from a woman with moderate hypertension. She has a strong family history of high blood pressure, and the regular practice of the Relaxation Response has lowered her blood pressure. She has been practicing the technique using the word "ONE" for over fourteen months. Her own words best convey what the response has meant to her.

The Relaxation Response has contributed to many changes in my life. Not only has it made me more relaxed physically and mentally, but also it has contributed to changes in my personality and way of life. I seem to have become calmer, more open and receptive especially to ideas which either have been unknown to me or very different from my past way of life. I like the way I am becoming; more patient, overcoming some fears especially around my physical health and stamina. I feel stronger physically and mentally. I take better care of myself. I am more committed to my daily exercise and see it as an integral part of my life. I really enjoy it, too! I drink less alcohol, take less medicine. The positive feedback which I experience as a result of the Relaxation Response and the lowered blood pressure readings make me feel I am attempting to transcend a family history replete with hypertensive heart disease.

I feel happier, content, and generally well when I use the Relaxation Response. There is a noticeable difference in attitude and energy during those occasional days in which I have had to miss the Relaxation Response.

Intellectually and spiritually, good things happen to me during the Relaxation Response. Sometimes I get insights into situations or problems which have been with me for a long time and about which I am not consciously thinking. Creative ideas come to me either during or as a direct result of the Relaxation Response. I look forward to the Relaxation Response twice and sometimes three times a day. I am hooked on it and love my addiction.

We should also comment about the side effects of the Relaxation Response. Any technique used to evoke the Relaxation Response trains you to let go of meaningful thoughts when they present themselves and to return to the repetition of the sound, the prayer, the word "ONE," or the mantra. Traditional psychoanalytic practice, on the other hand, trains you to hold on to free-association thoughts as working tools to open up your subconscious. Thus, there is a conflict between the methods of the Relaxation Response and those used in psychoanalysis. Persons undergoing psychoanalysis may have difficulty in disregarding distracting thoughts and assuming a passive attitude, and it may therefore be more difficult for them to elicit the Relaxation Response.

A basic teaching of many meditational organizations is that if a little meditation is good, a lot would be even better. This argument encourages followers to meditate for prolonged periods of time. From our personal observations, many people who meditate for several hours every day for weeks at a time tend to hallucinate. It is difficult, however, to draw a direct association between the Relaxation Response and this undesirable side effect because we do not know whether the people experiencing these side effects were predisposed to such problems to start with. For example, proponents of some meditative techniques evangelistically promise relief from all mental and physical suffering and tend to attract people who have emotional problems. There may be a preselection of people who come to learn these techniques because they already have emotional disturbances. Furthermore, the excessive daily elicitation of the Relaxation Response for many weeks may lead to hallucinations as a result of sensory deprivation. *We have not noted any of the above side effects in people who bring forth the Relaxation Response once or twice daily for ten to twenty minutes a day.*

One should not use the Relaxation Response in an effort to shield oneself or to withdraw from the pressures of the outside world which are necessary for everyday functioning. *The fight-or-flight response is often appropriate and should not be thought of as always harmful. It is a necessary part of our physiologic and psychological makeup, a useful reaction to many situations in our current world.* Modern society has forced us to evoke the fight-or-flight response repeatedly. We are not using it as we believe our ancestors used it. That is, we do not always run, nor do we fight when it is elicited. However, our body is being prepared for running or for fighting, and since this preparation is not always utilized, we believe anxieties, hypertension and its related diseases ensue. The Relaxation Response offers a natural balance to counteract the undesirable manifestations of the fight-or-flight response. We do not believe that you will become a passive and withdrawn person and less able to function and compete in our world because you regularly elicit the Relaxation Response. Rather, it has been our experience that people who regularly evoke the Relaxation Response claim they are more effective in dealing with situations that probably bring forth the fight-or-flight response. We believe you will be able to cope better with difficult situations by regularly allowing your body to achieve a more balanced state through the physiologic effects of the Relaxation Response. You can expect this balanced state to last as long as you regularly bring forth the response. Within several days after stopping its regular use, we believe, you will cease to benefit from its effects, *regardless* of the technique employed, be it prayer, Transcendental Meditation or the method proposed in this book.

8

·

Throughout this book we have tried to show you that the Relaxation Response is a natural gift that anyone can turn on and use. By bridging the traditional gaps between psychology, physiology, medicine, and history, we have established that the Relaxation Response is an innate mechanism within us.

The Relaxation Response is a universal human capacity, and even though it has been evoked in the religions of both East and West for most of recorded history, you don't have to engage in any rites or esoteric practices to bring it forth. The experience of the Relaxation Response has faded from our everyday life with the waning of religious practices and beliefs, but we can easily reclaim its benefits.

The people of the United States enjoy a standard of living and affluence beyond the experience of the majority of the world's people. But as individuals within this cornucopia, we are plagued by unhappiness. We seem never to be satisfied with what we have accomplished or what we possess. Perhaps it is ingrained in our present Western society that success and progress, no matter the price, are the names of the game. Go out, get as much as you can for yourself, don't be content with your present lot. The idealized work ethic reinforces the notion that monetary success or upward progression can be attained by a wide spectrum of our population. But even those who achieve these goals of monetary success and continued advancement are often not satisfied. They frequently find their lives thwarted by frustrating circumstances requiring behavioral adjustment. For those who do not advance in their careers or gain monetary security, behavioral adjustment is also necessary. Dissatisfaction, boredom, and unemployment should be looked upon as situations that require adjustment.

In most instances we cannot limit the situations that require behavioral adjustment. Because in our society we want more and we want it faster, this attitude does not leave time for relaxation or for appraising problems. When problems do develop, we look for a quick and easy solution. Our answer, aided by excessive advertising, is often to take a pill. You have only to turn on the television set and look at the advertising to see how we are trained to deal with problems. If you have tensions, pains, or insomnia, simply consume a tablet or capsule and your problems will disappear.

How can we thus deal with our anxieties and feelings of stress? Perhaps what we should do is modify our behavior by regularly evoking the Relaxation Response. If you view the Relaxation Response as a mechanism that effectively counters some of the harmful psychological and physiologic effects of our society, then the regular practice of the Relaxation Response may have an important place in your life. If you would regularly elicit this response, build it into your daily existence, the situations that activate your sympathetic nervous system could be counteracted by a process allowing your body to decrease its sympathetic nervous system activity. You would simply be using one innate body mechanism to counteract the effects of another.

Our Western society is oriented only in the direction of eliciting the fight-or-flight response. *Unlike the fight-or-flight response, which is repeatedly brought forth as a response to our difficult everyday situations and is elicited without conscious effort, the Relaxation Response can be evoked only if time is set aside and a conscious effort is made.* Our society has given very little attention to the importance of relaxation. Perhaps our work ethic views a person who takes time off as unproductive and lazy. At the same time, our society has eliminated many of the traditional methods of evoking the Relaxation Response. Prayer and meditation, as practiced by the ancients, have become part of our historical memory. We need the Relaxation Response even more today because our world is changing at an ever-increasing pace. Society should sanction the time for the Relaxation Response. Is it unreasonable to incorporate this inborn capacity into our daily lives by having a "Relaxation Response break" instead of a coffee break? You can choose any method of eliciting the response which best fits your own inclinations: a secular, a religious, or an Eastern technique. We could all greatly benefit by the reincorporation of the Relaxation Response into our daily lives. At the present time, most of us are simply not making use of this remarkable innate, neglected asset.

TO HELP YOU INCORPORATE
THE RELAXATION RESPONSE
IN YOUR DAILY LIFE, YOU MAY WISH TO
USE THIS CALENDAR

	Sun.	Mon.	Tues.
Week 1			
Week 2			
Week 3			
Week 4			
Week 5			

Make a check mark (✓) in the appropriate place

Wed.   Thurs.   Fri.   Sat.

each time you practice the Relaxation Response.

Bibliography

•

Abrahams, V.C.; Hilton, S. M.; and Zbrozyna, A. W. "Active Muscle Vasodilatation Produced by Stimulation of the Brain Stem: Its Significance in the Defense Reaction." *Journal of Physiology* 154 (1960): 491–513.

————. "The Role of Active Muscle Vasodilatation in the Altering Stage of the Defense Reaction." *Journal of Physiology* 171 (1964): 189–202.

Alexander, F. "Emotional Factors in Essential Hypertension. Presentation of a Tentative Hypothesis." *Psychosomatic Medicine* 1 (1939): 173–179.

Allison, J. "Respiration Changes During Transcendental Meditation." *Lancet* i (1970): 833–834.

Anand, B. K.; Chhina, G. S.; and Singh, B. "Some Aspects of Electroencephalographic Studies in Yogis." *Electroencephalography and Clinical Neurophysiology* 13 (1961): 452–456.

————. "Studies on Shri Ramananda Yogi During His Stay in an Air-tight Box." *Indian Journal of Medical Research* 49 (1961): 82–89.

Ashvagosha. *The Awakening of Faith*. Translated by T. Richard. London: Charles Skilton, 1961.

Astin, J. A. "Why Patients Use Alternative Medicine." *Journal of the American Medical Association* 279 (1998): 1548–1553.

Ayman, D. "The Personality Type of Patients with Arteriolar Essential Hypertension." *American Journal of the Medical Sciences* 186 (1933): 213–223.

Bagchi, B. K., and Wenger, M. A. "Electrophysiological Correlations of Some Yoga Exercises." *Electroencephalography and Clinical Neurophysiology* 7 (1957): 132–149.

Barber, T. X. "Physiological Effects of 'Hypnosis.'" *Psychological Bulletin* 58 (1961): 390–419.

Beary, J. F., and Benson, H. "A Simple Psychophysiologic Technique which Elicits the Hypometabolic Changes of the Relaxation Response." *Psychosomatic Medicine* 36 (1974): 115–120.

Becker, B. J. P. "Cardiovascular Disease in the Bantu and Coloured Races of South Africa." *South African Journal of Medical Sciences* 11 (1946): 107–120.

Beecher, H. "The Powerful Placebo." *Journal of the American Medical Association* 159 (1955): 1602–1606.

A Benedictine of Stanbrook Abbey. *Mediaeval Mystical Tradition and Saint John of the Cross.* London: Burns & Oates, 1954.

Benson, H. "Yoga for Drug Abuse." *New England Journal of Medicine* 281 (1969): 1133.

———. "Methods of Blood Pressure Recording: 1733 to 1971." In *Hypertension: Mechanisms and Management,* edited by G. Onesti; K. E. Kim; and J. H. Moyer, pp. 1– 8. New York: Grune and Stratton, 1973.

———. "Transcendental Meditation—Science or Cult?" *Journal of the American Medical Association* 227 (1974): 807.

———. "Your Innate Asset for Combatting Stress." *Harvard Business Review* 52 (1974): 49–60.

———. "Decreased Alcohol Intake Associated with the Practice of Meditation: A Retrospective Investigation." *Annals of the New York Academy of Sciences* 233 (1974): 174–177.

———. *Beyond the Relaxation Response.* New York: Times Books, 1984.

———. *Timeless Healing: The Power and Biology of Belief.* New York: Scribner, 1996.

Benson, H.; Beary, J. F.; and Carol, M. P. "The Relaxation Response." *Psychiatry* 37 (1974): 37–46.

Benson, H.; Costa, R.; Garcia-Palmieri, M. R.; Feliberti, M.; Aixala, R.; Blanton, J. A.; and Colon, A. A. "Coronary Heart Disease Risk Factors: A Comparison of Two Puerto Rican

Populations." *American Journal of Public Health and the Nation's Health* 56 (1966): 1057–1060.

Benson, H., and Dusek, J. A. "Self-Reported Health and Illness and the Use of Conventional and Unconventional Medicine and Mind/Body Healing by Christian Scientists and Others." *Journal of Nervous and Mental Disease* 187 (1999): 540–549.

Benson, H., and Friedman, R. "Harnessing the Power of the Placebo Effect and Renaming It 'Remembered Wellness.' " *Annual Review of Medicine* 47 (1996): 193–199.

Benson, H.; Greenwood, M. M.; and Klemchuk, H. P. "The Relaxation Response: Psychophysiologic Aspects and Clinical Applications." *Psychiatry in Medicine,* 6 (1975): 87–98.

Benson, H.; Herd, J. A.; Morse, W. H.; and Kelleher, R. T. "Behaviorally Induced Hypertension in the Squirrel Monkey." *Circulation Research Supplement* 1 26–27 (1970): 21–26.

Benson, H.; Herd, J. A.; Morse, W. H.; and Kelleher, R. T. "Behavioral Induction of Arterial Hypertension and its Reversal." *American Journal of Physiology* 217 (1969): 30–34.

Benson, H.; Klemchuk, H. P.; and Graham, J. R. "The Usefulness of the Relaxation Response in the Therapy of Headache." *Headache* 14 (1974): 49–52.

Benson, H.; Lehmann, J. W.; Malhotra, M. S.; Goldman, R. F.; Hopkins, J.; and Epstein, M. D. "Body Temperature Changes During the Practice of G Tum-Mo (Heat) Yoga." *Nature* 295 (1982): 234–236.

Benson, H.; Marzetta, B. R.; and Rosner, B. A. "Decreased Blood Pressure Associated with the Regular Elicitation of the Relaxation Response: A Study of Hypertensive Subjects." In *Con-*

temporary Problems in Cardiology, Vol. 1, *Stress and the Heart,* edited by R. S. Eliot, pp. 293–302. Mt. Kisco, New York: Futura, 1974.

————. "Decreased Systolic Blood Pressure in Hypertensive Subjects Who Practiced Meditation." *Journal of Clinical Investigation* 52 (1973): 8a.

Benson, H.; Rosner, B. A.; Marzetta, B. R.; and Klemchuk, H. P. "Decreased Blood Pressure in Pharmacologically Treated Hypertensive Patients Who Regularly Elicited the Relaxation Response." *Lancet* i (1974): 289–291.

————. "Decreased Blood Pressure in Borderline Hypertensive Subjects Who Practiced Meditation." *Journal of Chronic Diseases* 27 (1974): 163–169.

Benson, H.; Shapiro, D.; Tursky, B.; and Schwartz, G. E. "Decreased Systolic Blood Pressure through Operant Conditioning Techniques in Patients with Essential Hypertension." *Science* 173 (1971): 740–742.

Benson, H.; and Stuart, E.; Staff of the Mind/Body Medical Institute. *The Wellness Book.* New York: Carol, 1992.

Benson, H., and Wallace, R. K. "Decreased Drug Abuse with Transcendental Meditation—A Study of 1,862 Subjects." In *Drug Abuse—Proceedings of the International Conference,* edited by C. J. D. Zarafonetis, pp. 369–376. Philadelphia: Lea and Febiger, 1972.

Berkson, D. M.; Stamler, J.; Lindbergh, H. A.; Miller, W.; Mathias, H.; Lasky, H.; and Hall, Y. "Socioeconomic Correlates of Atherosclerotic and Hypertensive Heart Disease." *Annals of the New York Academy of Sciences* 84 (1960): 835–850.

Blair, D. A.; Glover, W. E.; Greenfield, A. D. M.; and Roddie, I. C. "The Activation of Cholinergic Vasodilator Nerves in the Human Forearm During Emotional Stress." *Journal of Physiology* 148 (1959): 633–647.

Bokser, Rabbi Ben Zion. *From the World of the Cabbalah.* New York: Philosophical Library, 1954.

Brebbia, D. R., and Altshuler, K. Z. "Oxygen Consumption Rate and Electroencephalographic Stage of Sleep." *Science* 150 (1965): 1621–1623.

Brod, J. "Essential Hypertension: Haemodynamic Observations with a Bearing on its Pathogenesis." *Lancet* ii (1960): 773–778.

———. "Haemodynamic Response to Stress and its Bearing on the Haemodynamic Basis of Essential Hypertension." In *The Pathogenesis of Essential Hypertension. Proceedings of the Prague Symposium,* edited by J. H. Cort, pp. 256–264. Prague: State Medical Publishing House, 1961.

———. "Circulation in Muscle During Acute Pressor Responses to Emotional Stress and During Chronic Sustained Elevation of Blood Pressure." *American Heart Journal* 68 (1964): 424–426.

Brod, J.; Fencl, V.; Hejl, Z.; and Jirka, J. "Circulatory Changes Underlying Blood Pressure Elevation During Acute Emotional Stress (Mental Arithmetic) in Normotensive and Hypertensive Subjects." *Clinical Science* 18 (1959): 269–279.

Brod, J.; Fencl, V.; Hejl, Z.; Jirka, J.; Ulrych, M. "General and Regional Haemodynamic Pattern Underlying Essential Hypertension." *Clinical Sciences* 23 (1962): 339–349.

Butler, C. *Western Mysticism.* London: Constable, 1922.

Cannon, W. B. "The Emergency Function of the Adrenal Medulla in Pain and the Major Emotions." *American Journal of Physiology* 33 (1914): 356–372.

———. *Bodily Changes in Pain, Hunger, Fear and Rage.* New York: Appleton, 1929.

———. *The Way of an Investigator. A Scientist's Experiences in Medical Research.* New York: W. W. Norton, 1945.

Chan, W. *A Source Book in Chinese Philosophy.* Princeton: Princeton University Press, 1963.

Chang, C.-Y. *Creativity and Taoism.* New York: Julian Press, 1963.

Christenson, W. N., and Hinkel, L. E. "Differences in Illness and Prognostic Signs in Two Groups of Young Men." *Journal of the American Medical Association* 177 (1961): 247–253.

The Cloud of Unknowing. Translated by Ira Progoff. New York: Dell Books, 1957.

Clynes, M. "Toward a View of Man." In *Biomedical Engineering Systems,* edited by M. Clynes and J. Milsum. New York: McGraw-Hill, 1970.

Cohen, M. E., and White, P. D. "Life Situations, Emotions and Neurocirculatory Asthenia (Anxiety Neurosis, Neurasthenia, Effort Syndrome)." *Research Publications of the Association for Research in Nervous and Mental Disease* 29 (1950): 832–869.

Crasilneck, H. B., and Hall, J. A. "Physiological Changes Associated with Hypnosis: A Review of the Literature Since 1948." *International Journal of Clinical and Experimental Hypnosis* 7 (1959): 9–50.

Cruz-Coke, R. "Environmental Influences and Arterial Blood Pressure." *Lancet* ii (1960): 885–886.

Dahl, L. K.; Knudson, K. D.; Heine, M.; and Leitl, G. "Hypertension and Stress." *Nature* 219 (1968): 735–736.

Datey, K. K.; Deshmukh, S. N.; Dalvi, C. P.; and Vinekar, S. L. " 'Shavasan': A Yogic Exercise in the Management of Hypertension." *Angiology* 20 (1969): 325–333.

Davis, R.C., and Kantor, J. R. "Skin Resistance During Hypnotic States." *Journal of General Psychology* 13 (1935): 62–81.

Dayton, S.; Pearce, M. L.; Hashimoto, S.; Dixon, W. J.; and Tomiyasu, U. "A Controlled Clinical Trial of a Diet High in Unsaturated Fat in Preventing Complications of Atherosclerosis." *Circulation* 40 (1969): 58–60.

Dean, S. R. "Is There an Ultraconscious Beyond the Unconscious?" *Canadian Psychiatric Association Journal* 15 (1970): 57–61.

Decker, D. G., and Rosenbaum, J. D. "The Distribution of Lactic Acid in Human Blood." *American Journal of Physiology* 138 (1942–43): 7–11.

Dudley, D. L.; Holmes, T. H.; Martin, C. J.; and Ripley, H. S. "Changes in Respiration Associated with Hypnotically Induced Emotion, Pain, and Exercise." *Psychosomatic Medicine* 26 (1963): 46–57.

Dykman, R. A., and Gantt, W. H. "Experimental Psychogenic Hypertension: Blood Pressure Changes Conditioned to Painful Stimuli (Schizokinesis)." *Bulletin of the Johns Hopkins Hospital* 107 (1960): 72–89.

Eich, R. H.; Cuddy, R. P.; Smulyan, H.; and Lyons, R. H. "Hae-modynamics in Labile Hypertension." *Circulation* 34 (1966): 299–307.

Eliade, M. *Yoga: Immortality and Freedom.* Translated by W. R. Trask. London: Routledge and Kegan Paul, 1958.

Estabrooks, G. H. "The Psychogalvanic Reflex in Hypnosis." *Journal of General Psychology* 3 (1930): 150–157.

Fischer, R. "A Cartography of the Ecstatic and Meditative States." *Science* 174 (1971): 897–904.

Folkow, B., and Rubinstein, E. H. "Cardiovascular Effects of Acute and Chronic Stimulations of the Hypothalamic Defense Area in the Rat." *Acta Physiologica Scandinavica* 68 (1966): 48–57.

Forsyth, R. P. "Blood Pressure and Avoidance Conditioning. A Study of 15-day Trials in the Rhesus Monkey." *Psychosomatic Medicine* 30 (1968): 125–135.

Friedman, E. H.; Hellerstein, H. K.; Eastwood, G. L.; and Jones, S. E. "Behavior Patterns and Serum Cholesterol in Two Groups of Normal Males." *American Journal of the Medical Sciences* 255 (1968): 237–244.

Friedman, M., and Rosenman, R. H. "Association of Specific Overt Behavior Pattern with Blood and Cardiovascular Findings." *Journal of the American Medical Association* 169 (1959): 1286–1296.

Frohlich, E. D.; Tarazi, R. C.; and Dustan, H. P. Reexamination of the Hemodynamics of Hypertension." *American Journal of the Medical Sciences* 257 (1969): 9–23.

Fujisawa, C. *Zen and Shinto*. New York: Philosophical Library, 1959.

Galbraith, J. K. *The Affluent Society*. New York: New American Library, 1958.

Gampel, M. B.; Slome, C.; Scotch, N.; and Abramson, J. H. "Urbanization and Hypertension among Zulu Adults." *Journal of Chronic Diseases* 15 (1962): 67–70.

Geiger, H. J., and Scotch, N. A. "The Epidemiology of Essential Hypertension. A Review with Special Attention to Psychologic and Sociocultural Factors. (1) Biologic Mechanisms and Descriptive Epidemiology." *Journal of Chronic Diseases* 16 (1963): 1151–1182.

Gellhorn, E. *Principles of Autonomic-Somatic Interactions*. Minneapolis: University of Minnesota Press, 1967.

Gellhorn, E., and Kiely, W. F. "Mystical States of Consciousness: Neurophysiological and Clinical Aspects." *Journal of Nervous and Mental Disease* 154 (1972): 399–405.

Glock, C. Y., and Lennard, H. L. "Studies in Hypertension. V. Psychologic Factors in Hypertension: An Interpretative Review." *Journal of Chronic Diseases* 5 (1957): 174–185.

Goldblatt, H.; Lynch, J.; Hanzal, R. F.; and Summerville, W. W. "Studies of Experimental Hypertension. I. The Production of Persistent Elevation of Systolic Blood Pressure by Means of Renal Ischemia." *Journal of Experimental Medicine* 59 (1934): 347–379.

Gordon, N. P.; Sobel, D. S., and Tarazona, E. Z. "Use of and Interest in Alternative Therapies Among Adult Primary Care

Clinicians and Adult Members in a Large Health Maintenance Organization." *Western Journal of Medicine* 169 (1998): 153–161.

Gordon, T., and Devine, B. "Hypertension and Hypertensive Heart Disease in Adults. Vital and Health Statistics." Washington, D. C.: Government Printing Office (PHS Publication No. 1000), 1966. pp. 1–11.

Gordon, T., and Waterhouse, A. M. "Hypertension and Hypertensive Heart Disease." *Journal of Chronic Diseases* 19 (1966): 1089–1100.

Gorton, B. E. "Physiology of Hypnosis." *Psychiatric Quarterly* 23 (1949): 317–343, 457–485.

Graham, J. D. P. "High Blood Pressure after Battle." *Lancet* 248 (1945): 239–240.

Grollman, A. "Physiological Variations in the Cardiac Output of Man." *American Journal of Physiology* 95 (1930): 274–284.

Grosz, H. J., and Farmer, B. B. "Pitts' and McClure's Lactate-Anxiety Study Revisited." *British Journal of Psychiatry* 120 (1972): 415–418.

Gutmann, M. C., and Benson, H. "Interaction of Environmental Factors and Systemic Arterial Blood Pressure: A Review." *Medicine* 50 (1971): 543–553.

Hamilton, J. A. "Psychophysiology of Blood Pressure. I. Personality and Behavior Ratings." *Psychosomatic Medicine* 4 (1942): 125–133.

Harburg, E.; Smedes, T.; Strauch, P.; Ward, L.; Nunce, R.; Stack, A.; and Donahue, K. "Progress Report: Stress and Heredity in Negro-White Blood Pressure Differences." United

States Public Health Service and Michigan Heart Association (HS 00164–05), January, 1970. pp. 1–26.

Harris, R. E., and Singer, M. T. "Interaction of Personality and Stress in the Pathogenesis of Essential Hypertension." *Hypertension, Proceedings of the Council of High Blood Pressure Research* 16 (1967): 104–115.

Harris, R. E.; Sokolow, M.; Carpenter, L. B.; Freedman, M.; and Hunt, S. P. "Response to Psychologic Stress in Persons Who are Potentially Hypertensive." *Circulation* 7 (1953): 874–879.

Hart, J. T. "Autocontrol of EEG Alpha." *Psychophysiology* 4 (1968): 506.

Hawkins, D. R.; Puryeur, H. B.; Wallace, C. D.; Deal, W. B.; and Thomas, E. S. "Basal Skin Resistance during Sleep and 'Dreaming.' " *Science* 136 (1962): 321–322.

Henry, J. P., and Cassel, J. C. "Psychosocial Factors in Essential Hypertension. Recent Epidemiologic and Animal Experimental Evidence." *American Journal of Epidemiology* 90 (1969): 171–200.

Henry, J. P.; Meehan, J. P.; and Stephens, P. M. "The Use of Psychosocial Stimuli to Induce Prolonged Systolic Hypertension in Mice." *Psychosomatic Medicine* 29 (1967): 408–432.

Herbert, J. *Shinto; at the Fountain-head of Japan.* London: Allen and Unwin, 1967.

Herd, J. A.; Morse, W. H.; Kelleher, R. T.; and Jones, T. G. "Arterial Hypertension in the Squirrel Monkey During Behavioral Experiments." *American Journal of Physiology* 217 (1969): 24–29.

Hess, W. R. *The Functional Organization of the Diencephalon.* New York: Grune and Stratton, 1957.

Hess, W. R., and Brugger, M. "Das Subkortikale Zentrum der Affektiven Abwehrreaktion." *Helvetica Physiologica et Pharmacologica Acta* 1 (1943): 33–52.

Heymans, C.; Bouckaert, L.; and Dautrebande, L. "Sur la Regulation Reflexe de la Circulation par les Nerfs Vasosensibles du Sinus Carotidien." *Archives Internationales de Pharmacodynamie et de Therapie* 40 (1931): 292–343.

Hilton, S. M. "Hypothalamus Regulation of the Cardiovascular System." *British Medical Bulletin* 22 (1966): 243–248.

Hinkle, L. E., and Wolff, G. E. "The Role of Emotional and Environmental Factors in Essential Hypertension." In *The Pathogenesis of Essential Hypertension. Proceedings of the Prague Symposium,* edited by J. H. Cort, pp. 129–143. Prague: State Medical Publishing House, 1961.

Hoenig, J. "Medical Research on Yoga." *Confinia Psychiatrica* II (1968): 69–89.

Holmes, T. H., and Rahe, R. H. "The Social Readjustment Rating Scale." *Journal of Psychosomatic Research* 11 (1967): 213.

Huang Ti Nei Ching Su Wên. The Yellow Emperor's Classic of Internal Medicine. Translated by Ilza Veith. Berkeley: University of California Press, 1966.

Ishiguro, H. *The Scientific Truth of Zen.* Tokyo: Zenrigaku Society, 1964.

Jacobson, E. *Progresssive Relaxation.* Chicago: University of Chicago Press, 1938.

James, W. *Letters*. Boston: Atlantic Monthly Press, 1920.

———. *The Varieties of Religious Experience*. New York: New American Library, 1958.

Jana, H. "Energy Metabolism in Hypnotic Trance and Sleep." *Journal of Applied Physiology* 20 (1965): 308–310.

———. "Effect of Hypnosis on Circulation and Respiration." *Indian Journal of Medical Research* 55 (1967): 591–598.

Jenkins, C. D.; Rosenman, R. H.; and Friedman, M. "Development of an Objective Psychological Test for the Determination of the Coronary-Prone Behavior Pattern in Employed Men." *Journal of Chronic Diseases* 20 (1967): 371–379.

John of Ruysbroeck. *The Adornment of the Spiritual Alphabet*. Translated by C. A. Wynschenk. London: J.M. Dent & Sons, 1916.

Johnson, R. C. *Watcher on the Hills*. New York: Harper and Brothers, 1959.

Johnston, W. *Christian Zen*. New York: Harper & Row, 1971.

Jones, M., and Mellersh, V. "Comparison of Exercise Response in Anxiety States and Normal Controls." *Psychosomatic Medicine* 8 (1946): 180–187.

Kalis, B.; Harris, R.; Bennett, L. F.; and Sokolow, M. "Personality and Life History Factors in Persons Who Are Potentially Hypertensive." *Journal of Nervous and Mental Disease* 132 (1961): 457–468.

Kamiya, J. "Operant Control of the EEG Alpha Rhythm and Some of Its Reported Effects on Consciousness." In *Altered States of Consciousness*, edited by C. T. Tart, pp. 507–517. New York: John Wiley & Sons, 1969.

Kannel, W. B.; Dawber, T. R.; Kagan, A.; and Revotskie, N. "Factors of Risk in the Development of Coronary Heart Disease—Six Year Follow-up Experience." *Annals of Internal Medicine* 55 (1961): 33–50.

Kannel, W. B.; Schwartz, M. J.; and McNamara, P. M. "Blood Pressure and Risk of Coronary Heart Disease: The Framingham Study." *Diseases of the Chest* 56 (1969): 43–52.

Karambelkar, P. V.; Vinekar, S. L.; and Bhole, M. V. "Studies on Human Subjects Staying in an Air-tight Pit." *Indian Journal of Medical Research* 56 (1968): 1282–1288.

Kasamatsu, A., and Hirai, T. "An Electroencephalographic Study on the Zen Meditation (Zazen)." *Folia Psychiatrica et Neurologica Japonica* 20 (1966): 315–336.

Kass, E. H., and Zinner, S. H. "How Early Can the Tendency Toward Hypertension be Detected?" *Milbank Memorial Fund Quarterly* 47 (1969): 143–152.

Katkin, H. S., and Murray, E. N. "Instrumental Conditioning of Autonomically Mediated Behavior: Theoretical and Methodological Issues." *Psychological Bulletin* 70 (1968): 52–68.

Keith, R. L.; Lown, B.; and Stare, F. J. "Coronary Heart Disease and Behavior Patterns." *Psychosomatic Medicine* 27 (1965): 424–434.

Kezdi, P. "Etiologic Mechanisms in Prehypertension." *Current Theory of Research and Clinical Experimentation* 5 (1963): 553–563.

———. "Neurogenic Control of the Blood Pressure in Hypertension." *Cardiologia* 51 (1967): 193–203.

Kleitman, N. *Sleep and Wakefulness*. Chicago: University of Chicago Press, 1963.

Kreider, M. B., and Iampietro, P. F. "Oxygen Consumption and Body Temperature During Sleep in Cold Environments." *Journal of Applied Physiology* 14 (1959): 765–767.

Kroenke, K., and Mangelsdorff, A. D. "Common Symptoms in Ambulatory Care: Incidence, Evaluation, Therapy and Outcome." *American Journal of Medicine* 86 (1989): 262–266.

Langford, H. G.; Watson, R. L.; and Douglas, B. H. "Factors Affecting Blood Pressure in Population Groups." *Transactions of the Association of American Physicians* 81 (1968): 135–146.

Lapin, B. A. "Response of the Cardiovascular System of Monkeys to Stress." *Acta Cardiologica* II (1965): 276–280.

Laragh, J. H. "Recent Advances in Hypertension." *American Journal of Medicine* 39 (1965): 616–645.

Lennard, H. L., and Glock, C. Y. "Studies in Hypertension. VI. Differences in the Distribution of Hypertension in Negroes and Whites; An Appraisal." *Journal of Chronic Diseases* 5 (1957): 186–196.

Levander, V. L.; Benson, H.; Wheeler, R. C.; and Wallace, R. K. "Increased Forearm Blood Flow During a Wakeful Hypometabolic State." *Federation Proceedings* 31 (1972): 405.

Levene, H. I.; Engel, B. T.; and Pearson, J. A. "Differential Operant Conditioning of Heart Rate." *Psychosomatic Medicine* 30 (1968): 837–845.

Levine, S. A. "Angina Pectoris in Father and Son." *American Heart Journal* 66 (1963): 49–52.

Louis, W. J.; Doyle, A. E.; and Anavekar, S. "Plasma Norepinephrine Levels in Essential Hypertension." *New England Journal of Medicine* 288 (1973): 599–601.

Lowell, P. *The Soul of the Far East.* Boston: Houghton Mifflin, 1892.

Luthe, W., ed. *Autogenic Therapy.* Vols. 1–5. New York: Grune and Stratton, 1969.

Maddocks, I. "The Influence of Standard of Living on Blood Pressure in Fiji." *Circulation* 24 (1961): 1220–1223.

Maharishi Mahesh Yogi. *The Science of Being and Art of Living.* London: International SRM Publications, 1966.

Marzetta, B. R.; Benson, H.; and Wallace, R. K. "Combatting Drug Dependency in Young People; A New Approach." *Counterpoint* 4 (1972): 13–36.

Miall, W. E.; Kass, E. H.; Ling, J.; and Stuart, K. L. "Factors Influencing Arterial Pressure in the General Population in Jamaica." *British Medical Journal* 2 (1962): 497–506.

Miall, W. E., and Oldham, P. D. "Factors Influencing Arterial Blood Pressure in the General Population." *Clinical Science* 17 (1958): 409–444.

Miller, N. E. "Learning of Visceral and Glandular Responses." *Science* 163 (1969): 434–445.

Molen, R. V.; Brewer, G.; Honeyman, M. F.; Morrison, J.; and Hoobler, S. W. "A Study of Hypertensive Twins." *American Heart Journal* 79 (1970): 454–457.

Naranjo, C., and Ornstein, R. E. *On the Psychology of Meditation.* New York: Viking Press, 1971.

Needleman, J. *The New Religions*. Garden City, N.Y.: Doubleday, 1970.

NIH Technology Assessment Panel on Integration of Behavioral and Relaxation Approaches into the Treatment of Chronic Pain and Insomnia. *Journal of the American Medical Association* 276 (1996): 313–318.

Norwich, J. J., and Sitwell, R. *Mount Athos*. New York: Harper & Row, 1966.

Organ, T. W. *The Hindu Quest for the Perfection of Man*. Athens, Ohio: Ohio University Press, 1970.

Ornstein, R. E. *The Psychology of Consciousness*. San Francisco: W. H. Freeman, 1972.

Ostfeld, A. M., and Lebovits, B. Z. "Personality Factors and Pressor Mechanisms in Renal and Essential Hypertension." *Archives of Internal Medicine* 104 (1959): 43–52.

———. "Blood Pressure Lability: A Correlative Study." *Journal of Chronic Diseases* 12 (1960): 428–439.

Ostfeld, A. M., and Shekelle, R. B. "Psychological Variables and Blood Pressure." In *The Epidemiology of Hypertension,* edited by J. Stamler; R. Stamler; and T. N. Pullman, pp. 321–331. New York: Grune and Stratton, 1967.

Osuna, F. F. D. *The Third Spiritual Alphabet*. New York: Benziger Brothers, 1931.

Otto, R. *Mysticism East and West: A Comparative Analysis of the Nature of Mysticism*. New York: Macmillan, 1932.

Palmer, R. S. "Psyche and Blood Pressure. One Hundred Mental Stress Tests and Fifty Personality Surveys in Patients with

Essential Hypertension." *Journal of the American Medical Association* 144 (1950): 295–298.

Patel, C. H. "Yoga and Biofeedback in the Management of Hypertension." *Lancet* ii (1973): 1053–1055.

————. "12–Month Follow-up of Yoga and Biofeedback in the Management of Hypertension." *Lancet* i (1975): 62–64.

Pitts, F. N., Jr., and McClure, J. N., Jr. "Lactate Metabolism in Anxiety Neurosis." *New England Journal of Medicine* 277 (1967): 1329–1336.

Rahe, R. H. "Subjects' Recent Life Changes and Their Near-Future Illness Reports." *Annals of Clinical Research* 4 (1972): 250–265.

Ramamurthi, B. "Yoga: An Explanation and Probable Neurophysiology." *Journal of the Indian Medical Association* 48 (1967): 167–170.

Reschtschaffen, A.; Kales, A.; Berger, R. J.; Dement, W. C.; Jacobson, A.; Johnson, L. C.; Jouvet, M.; Monroe, L. J.; Oswald, I.; Roffward, H. P.; Roth, B.; and Walter, R. D. *A Manual of Standardized Terminology, Technique and Scoring System for Sleep Stages of Human Subjects*. Washington, D.C.: U.S. Government Printing Office (Public Health Service), 1968.

Rierenbaum, M. L.; Fleischman, A. I.; Raichelson, R. I.; Hayton, T.; Watson, P. B. "Ten-Year Experience of Modified-Fat Diets on Younger Men with Coronary Heart Disease." *Lancet* i (1973): 1404–1407.

Robbins, P. R. "Personality and Psychosomatic Illness: A Selective Review of Research." *Genetic Psychology Monographs* 80 (1969): 51–90.

Roberts, A. H.; Kewman, D. G.; Mercier, L.; and Hovell, M. "The Power of Nonspecific Effects in Healing: Implications for Psychosocial and Biological Treatments." *Clinical Psychology Review* 13 (1993): 375–391.

Robin, E. D.; Whaley, R. D.; Crump, C. H.; and Travis, D. M. "Alveolar Gas Tensions, Pulmonary Ventilation and Blood pH During Physiologic Sleep in Normal Subjects." *Journal of Clinical Investigation* 37 (1958): 981–989.

Rosenman, R. H., and Friedman, M. "Behavior Patterns, Blood Lipids, and Coronary Heart Disease. *Journal of the American Medical Association* 184 (1963): 934–938.

Rosenman, R. H.; Friedman, M.; Straus, R.; Wurm, M.; Jenkins, D.; and Messinger, H. "Coronary Heart Disease in the Western Collaborative Group Study." *Journal of the American Medical Association* 195 (1966): 86–92.

Rosenman, R. H.; Friedman, M.; Straus, R.; Wurm, M.; Kositechek, R.; Hahn, W.; and Werthessen, N. T. "A Predictive Study of Coronary Heart Disease." *Journal of the American Medical Association* 189 (1964): 15–22.

Ross, F. H. *Shinto, The Way of Japan*. Boston: Beacon Press, 1965.

Ross, R., and Glomset, J. A. "Atherosclerosis and the Arterial Smooth Muscle Cell." *Science* 180 (1973): 1332–1339.

Rousch, W. "Herbert Benson: Mind-Body Maverick Pushes the Envelope." *Science* 276 (1997): 357–359.

Rushmer, R. F. *Cardiovascular Dynamics*. Philadelphia: W. B. Saunders, 1961.

Ruskin, A.; Beard, O. W.; and Schaffer, R. L. "Blast Hypertension. Elevated Arterial Pressures in the Victims of the Texas City Disaster." *American Journal of Medicine* 4 (1948): 228–236.

Saddhatissa, H. *The Buddha's Way.* London: Allen and Unwin, 1971.

St. Augustine. *The Confessions of St. Augustine.* Translated by E. B. Pusey. London: Everyman's Library. 1966.

Saint Teresa of Jesus. *The Way of Perfection.* Translated by A. D. Carmelite. Edinborough: Joseph Leighton, 1941.

Sanborn, F. B. *Familiar Letters of Henry David Thoreau.* Boston: Houghton Mifflin, 1894.

Scholem, G. G. *Jewish Mysticism.* New York: Schocken Books, 1967.

Scotch, N. A. "Sociocultural Factors in the Epidemiology of Zulu Hypertension." *American Journal of Public Health and the Nation's Health* 53 (1963): 1205–1213.

Scotch, N.A., and Geiger, H. J. "The Epidemiology of Essential Hypertension. A Review with Special Attention to Psychologic and Sociocultural Factors. (II) Psychologic and Sociocultural Factors in Etiology." *Journal of Chronic Diseases* 16 (1963): 1183–1213.

Segal, J., ed. *Mental Health Program Report: 5.* Washington, D.C.: National Institute of Public Health, 1971.

Selye, H. *Stress without Distress.* Philadelphia: J. B. Lippincott, 1974.

Senate Rpt. 105–300. Departments of Labor, Health and Human Services, and Education and Related Agencies Appropriation

Bill. Office of the Director. Office of Behavioral and Social Sciences Research. (Associated Bill S. 2440). 1999.

Shapiro, A. P., and Horn, P. W. "Blood Pressure, Plasma Pepsinogen, and Behavior in Cats Subjected to Experimental Production of Anxiety." *Journal of Nervous and Mental Disease* 122 (1955): 222–231.

Shapiro, D.; Schwartz, G. E.; and Benson, H. "Biofeedback: A Behavioral Approach to Cardiovascular Self-Control." In *Contemporary Problems in Cardiology,* Vol. 1, *Stress and the Heart,* edited by R. S. Eliot, pp. 279–292. Mt. Kisco, New York: Futura, 1974.

Shapiro, D.; Tursky, B.; Gershon, E.; and Stern, M. "Effects of Feedback and Reinforcement on the Control of Human Systolic Blood Pressure." *Science* 163 (1969): 588–590.

Shiomi, K. "Respiratory and EEG Changes by Contention of Trigent Burrow." *Psychologia* 12 (1969): 24–28.

Simonson, E., and Brozek, J. "Russian Research on Arterial Hypertension." *Annals of Internal Medicine* 50 (1959): 129–193.

Skinner, B. F. *Science and Human Behavior.* New York: Macmillan, 1953.

Sokolow, M.; Kalis, B. L.; Harris, R. E.; and Bennett, L. F. "Personality and Predisposition to Essential Hypertension." In *The Pathogenesis of Essential Hypertension. Proceedings of the Prague Symposium,* edited by J. H. Cort, pp. 143–153. Prague: State Medical Publishing House, 1961.

Spurgeon, C. F. E. *Mysticism in English Literature.* Port Washington: Kennikat Press, 1970.

Stamler, J.; Berkson, D. M.; Lindberg, H. A.; Miller, W. A.; Stamler, R.; and Collette, P. "Socioeconomic Factors in the Epidemiology of Hypertensive Disease." In *The Epidemiology of Hypertension,* edited by J. Stamler; R. Stamler; and T. N. Pullman, pp. 289–313. New York: Grune and Stratton, 1967.

Sugi, Y., and Akutsu, K. "Studies on Respiration and Energy-Metabolism During Sitting in Zazen." *Research Journal of Physical Education* 12 (1968): 190–206.

Syme, S. L.; Hyman, M. M.; and Enterline, P. E. "Some Social and Cultural Factors Associated with the Occurrence of Coronary Heart Disease." *Journal of Chronic Diseases* 17 (1964): 277–289.

"Sympathetic Activity in Essential Hypertension" (editorial). *New England Journal of Medicine* 288 (1973): 627–629.

Tart, C. T. "Patterns of Basal Skin Resistance During Sleep." *Psychophysiology* 4 (1967): 35–39.

Thomas, C. B. "The Psychological Dimensions of Hypertension." In *The Epidemiology of Hypertension,* edited by J. Stamler; R. Stamler; and T. N. Pullman, pp. 332–339. New York: Grune and Stratton, 1967.

Thoreau, H. D. *Walden.* Princeton, N.J.: Princeton University Press, 1971.

Toffler, A. *Future Shock.* New York: Random House, 1970.

"Transcendental Meditation" (editorial). *Lancet* i (1972): 1058–1059.

Triminham, J. S. *Sufi Orders in Islam.* Oxford: Clarendon Press, 1971.

Tucker, W. I. "Psychiatric Factors in Essential Hypertension." *Diseases of the Nervous System* 10 (1949): 273–278.

Underhill, E. *Mysticism*. London: Methuen, 1957.

United States Department of Health, Education, and Welfare, Vital and Health Statistics. *Mortality Trends for Leading Causes of Death* (DHEW) Publication No. [HRA] 74–1853. Series 20. No. 16. Washington, D.C.: Government Printing Office, 1974.

Uvnas, B. "Cholinergic Vasodilator Nerves." *Federation Proceedings* 25 (1966): 1618–1622.

Valentin, J. *The Monks of Mt. Athos*. Translated by D. Athill. London: Andre Deutsch, 1960.

Veterans Administration Cooperative Study Group on Antihypertensive Agents. "Effects of Treatment on Morbidity in Hypertension. I. Results in Patients with Diastolic Blood Pressures Averaging 115 Through 129 mm Hg." *Journal of the American Medical Association* 202 (1967): 1028–1034.

Veterans Administration Cooperative Study Group on Antihypertensive Agents. "Effects of Treatment on Morbidity in Hypertension. II. Results in Patients with Diastolic Blood Pressure Averaging 90 Through 114 mm Hg." *Journal of the American Medical Association* 213 (1970): 1143–1152.

Wallace, R. K. "Physiological Effects of Transcendental Meditation." *Science* 167 (1970): 1751–1754.

Wallace, R. K., and Benson, H. "The Physiology of Meditation." *Scientific American* 226 (1972): 84–90.

Wallace, R. K.; Benson, H.; and Wilson, A. F. "A Wakeful Hypo-metabolic Physiologic State." *American Journal of Physiology* 221 (1971): 795–799.

Wallace, R. K.; Benson, H.; Wilson, A. F.; and Garrett, M. D. "Decreased Blood Lactate During Transcendental Medita-tion." *Federation Proceedings* 30 (1971): 376.

Weitzenhoffer, A. M., and Hilgard, E. *Stanford Hypnotic Suggest-ibility Scale*. Palo Alto: Consulting Psychologists Press, 1959.

Wenger, M. A.; Bagchi, B. K.; and Anand, B. K. "Experiments in India on 'Voluntary' Control of the Heart and Pulse." *Cir-culation* 24 (1961): 1319–1325.

Wheelis, A. *The Quest for Identity*. New York: W. W. Norton, 1958.

Whitehorn, J. C.; Lundholm, H.; Fox, E. L.; and Benedict, F. G. "The Metabolic Rate in Hypnotic Sleep." *New England Jour-nal of Medicine* 206 (1932): 777–781.

Zwemer, S. M. *A Moslem Seeker after God*. New York: Fleming H. Revell, 1920.

Index

•

Relaxation Response *cont.*
 physiologic changes associated
  with, (Fig. 9) 54, 75–76,
  109, 111–18, 128
 schools and universities, intro-
  duction in, li
 side effects of, 136–37
Relaxation therapy, 73–74
 autogenic training, 74, 75
 hypnosis with suggested deep relaxation, 74, 75, 77
 progressive, 74, 75, 77
Religion, 82–85
 See also Contemplation, Mysticism, Prayer
Remembered wellness, xxix, xxx
Respiration rate, 71, 75, 115
Retroprospective studies, 45
Reverence, 78
Rheumatoid arthritis, xlii
Rockefeller, Laurance, xxx
Rosner, B. A., 112
Rubinstein, E. H., 50

S
Saddhatissa, H., 100–101
Scale of stressful events, 39–40
Scholem, Gershom G., 97
Self-care, xii, xxxiii–xxxiv, xli,
  xliii–xliv
Selye, Hans, 37
Sentic cycles, 74, 75, 78
Sex, 78
Shamanism, 106
Shekelle, R. B., 44
Shelley, Maynard W., 122
Shultz, H. H., 74
Skinner, B. F., 56
Sleep, 86, 132

 meditation vs., 65–72
Sleeping pills, 132
Smoking, 119, 121
 heart disease and, 25
Social readjustment scale, 38
Spurgeon, Carolyn, 99, 106
Stark, Mark, xx
STP, 120
Stress, xiv, 1–2, 37–41, 124, 142
 change, adjusting to, 3, 39–40
 emotional, 37
 environmental, 6, 37, 41
 fight-or-flight response. *See*
  Fight-or-flight response
 hypertension and, xiii–xiv, xv,
  6–7, 35
 internal signs of, 47–54
 physiological, 37
 physiology of, 4
 scale of stressful events, 39–40
 victims of, 2–4
Stress management, xii
Strokes, 4–6, 11, 14, 22, 24, 31, 116
Studies
 blood pressure, decreasing,
  112–15, 117
 drug abuse, decreasing, 118–23
 prospective, 46
 retroprospective, 45
Surgery, xii, xxiii
Sympathetic nervous system, 52,
  72, 115, 142
Systolic blood pressure, 22, (Fig.
  5) 23

T
Taosim, 104–6
Templeton, Sir John, xxx
Tennyson, Alfred, 107, 109